OVERDUE

Quality Care for Our Elder Citizens

Phyllis Ayman

HybridGlobal
PUBLISHING

Published by
Hybrid Global Publishing
301 E 57th Street, 4th fl
New York, NY 10022

Manufactured in the United States of America, or in the United Kingdom when distributed elsewhere.

Ayman, Phyllis
    Overdue: Quality Care for Our Elder Citizens
    LCCN: 2019931420
    ISBN: 978-1-948181-42-6
    eBook: 978-1-948181-43-3

Cover design by: Joe Potter
Interior design: Claudia Volkman

Publicity is justly commended as a remedy for social and industrial diseases. Sunlight is said to be the best of disinfectants.
JUSTICE LOUIS D. BRANDEIS

DEDICATION

This book is dedicated to all of our elder citizens.
They all matter.

ACKNOWLEDGMENTS

This book could not have been published without Karen Strauss from Global Hybrid Publishing. Karen stepped in at the eleventh hour, on the recommendation from my business strategist Christopher Salem. Her support, guidance, and results-oriented approach was just what I needed at the time.

Claudia Volkman, my editor, worked indefatigably to complete the process in a matter of weeks when it usually takes months. She worked on holidays, weekends, and evenings to ensure we could meet the deadline. She made it easy and effortless. Claudia, I can't thank you enough.

Christopher Salem, my business strategist whose tireless effort, support, advice, guidance, and professionalism are second to none, was by my side throughout the entire process, and I couldn't have done it without him. Christopher, I am so appreciative and grateful that we are working together. The value you bring exceeds all expectations.

Bob Still of Still Digital Studios created my banners and logo. His generous spirit and all around good guy nature was evident in the many conversations we had. He took the time to understand my point of view which, combined with his artistic vision and talent, brought my concepts to life in a way I never could have imagined.

As always, my friend, teacher and mentor Suzanne Swope, was there to guide, reread, listen, and help me focus my ideas for pinpoint accuracy. Her observations are nothing short of brilliant.

There are no words to express my gratitude to Charlene Harrington, who agreed to write the foreword. I am so proud to have her lend her name to this book.

Finally, thanks to my friends and colleagues who consistently encouraged me in this process by reminding me of the importance and need for this work.

CONTENTS

FOREWORD

As a researcher studying nursing homes, I have been writing about nursing home problems for more years than I care to remember. During that time, nursing homes have made some improvements, but resident care continues to be substandard in many of our nation's nursing homes. Problems with insufficient nurse staffing are widespread, which in turn is related to poor resident care, such as the continued overuse of antipsychotic drugs, falls, pressure ulcers, weight loss, depression, rehospitalization, other negative consequences, and even death. These staffing and quality problems are occurring as nursing home residents have higher care needs than ever before.

Even more problematic is the proliferation of nursing home chains and corporations that are buying up smaller, independent and not-for-profit facilities in an effort to amass large profits. Research shows that for-profit nursing homes and chains have the lowest nurse staffing and the most quality of care problems. Ultimately, the care of the residents in many for-profit facilities continues to suffer.

Phyllis began writing a book in an effort to provide information to individuals and families who are considering entering a nursing home. As a speech pathologist who has worked in over forty nursing homes over twenty-five years, Phyllis has struggled to advocate for improved care and a range of programs to improve the quality of life for residents. Although a dedicated professional, she wanted to step outside of the daily work environment where she admittedly derived great satisfaction from making a difference in the lives of residents. She has likened the hurdles and challenges of nursing home work to a fish swimming upstream against indomitable currents leading to increasing frustration and exhaustion. This became the impetus for her taking a giant step to make a larger impact by informing people about nursing home care so they could become more effective advocates for themselves and their loved ones.

With her second book on nursing home care, Phyllis continues to express her passion for care rooted in her personal experience. In taking on this book, she has become an effective "voice for eldercare advocacy." She is speaking for those who cannot speak for themselves. Phyllis has shown herself to have a thorough command of the issues, and she is a creative thinker, good researcher, and effective communicator.

For those of us who have been involved in systemic advocacy, it is refreshing to hear from someone with a unique voice based on professional experience working within the nursing home industry. Phyllis has the hands-on knowledge of how nursing home care affects the lives of residents as well as their family and friends. More important, she has determination, dedication, courage, and heart to write about how care can be improved for the 1.5 million nursing home residents in the US. This book sheds light on care issues that need to be addressed and the policies and practices that need to be changed to ensure the best of care for all those in need.

—Charlene Harrington, PhD, RN Professor Emeritus
Department of Social & Behavioral Sciences
University of California San Francisco

PROLOGUE

It was 1974, and I was fifteen years old living in Brooklyn, New York. My grandmother had become increasingly frail and her care needs intensified. My mother made a valiant attempt to care for her several times a week, traveling the hour and a half by bus and train from Brooklyn to the Bronx. The long trip eventually took a toll on her. Grandma's physical condition deteriorated, and the family was forced to make a decision that no one ever really wants to have to make—not then, not now—to put her in a nursing home. In our case, thankfully, it was a few blocks from where we lived.

My mother walked the five or six blocks to this small nursing home every day. She went there first thing in the morning with clean clothes and a nutrient rich eggnog drink in tow, and she remained throughout the day until she was able to see that my grandmother was safely in bed and asleep. It would be about 9:00 p.m. when she finally arrived home. This continued for approximately a year before my grandmother passed away.

My grandmother was an extremely proud and pristine woman who couldn't stand the thought of anyone seeing her use a walker, which she needed after she broke her hip and her Parkinson's disease progressed. That's why the horrific scene I encountered the first time I went to see her in the nursing home was that much more difficult to bear.

I walked up to the entrance and opened the front door. The lobby had an overwhelming stench that assaulted my nostrils. But worse than the nauseating smell was what I first saw. There was my grandmother, that wonderful woman I knew and adored, sitting slumped in a wheelchair with copious amounts of saliva drooling from her mouth onto her clothes. Overwhelmed by the sight, I turned around and ran out the door, hoping Grandma didn't see me. I just could not deal with what I saw! After walking around the block several times with tears streaming down my face, I finally mustered enough courage to go back in and attend to Grandma's needs. After all, that was what I came to do, and that was more important than how I felt about it at the moment. What could I do to help her maintain more of the dignity she deserved? This experience left an indelible mark on my mind and heart and has stayed with me until this day.

At one point during the year my parents went away for a two-week vacation to celebrate their twenty-fifth wedding anniversary. During that time, my sister and I took turns each day to care for my grandmother in my mother's absence. My sister, who was in college, took the morning shift before her scheduled afternoon classes. I, being a high schooler, took the afternoon shift after getting home from school.

On Mother's Day 1969, my uncle, who was my mother's brother, and his wife came with their two daughters to see my grandmother and spend some time with my sister and me. My uncle went to see his mother, but my aunt would not go, nor would she allow her daughters to visit their grandmother, one of whom was a teenager older than me, the other a year younger. I'll never forget what she said to me as we stood on the sunbaked front porch of our house on that beautiful sunny Sunday. She said it was "too depressing." She did not want to go into an "old age home and see what happens to old people." *Old people*—the very people who fed and clothed us, nurtured us, and helped us grow up.

Furthermore, she wondered how my sister and I could stand to be doing this. I told her that I was glad to do it, first out of respect for my mother and her respect for hers. But I also told my aunt that it would help me to understand what it was like to become old, to not be afraid of it, and it would help me know how to take care of my mother when she approached that time.

Circumstances were such that I did not have that opportunity with my mother; however, I believe the experience with my grandmother helped shape the course of my professional life.

Years later, after becoming a speech pathologist, I felt the urge to return the nursing home environment so I could specialize in caring for our elders, hopefully providing something better than what my grandmother experienced.

The stories included in this book are firsthand accounts of my personal experiences and/or experiences of my colleagues. I chose them to reflect the problematic issues related to nursing homes and rehabilitation centers, how these issues can impact care decisions and the quality of care provided. The stories are set apart from the chapter information by their descriptive titles and distinctive print.

PART ONE

THE STATE OF ELDERCARE IN AMERICA

ONE

WE *CAN* DO BETTER

FORTY YEARS OF FIGHTING FOR RESPECT AND DECENT ELDERCARE

In 1978 Mrs. Margaret Maunder was president of Healthpower of Hamden, Connecticut, a healthcare agency that provided assistance for elder citizens. Forty years ago, she presented an award to Grace Lenox Flight, a licensed nursing home administrator and director of education at Bentley Gardens Nursing Home in West Haven, Connecticut. Ms. Flight was distinguished for her efforts as founder of the Committee on Geriatric Nursing Education, a voluntary group of four hundred nurses in the state of Connecticut working to improve the quality of healthcare for elder citizens.

It's truly a remarkable story.

I had become friends with a woman I met at a mutual friend's house. Initially our conversation was limited to the movies our friend showed to the friends who gathered at his house on Sunday evenings, but we soon found we had other similar interests.

One particular evening, the conversation came around to the topic of nursing homes, as it was shortly after my first book, *Nursing Homes to Rehabilitation Centers: What Every Person Needs to Know,* had been published. My friend proceeded to tell me that her mother had been in a nursing home in another state up until her death the year before. The stories she told me when she went to visit her mom were all too familiar: short staff, poor quality of care, poor attitude in general, poor food quality, and less than optimally clean surroundings. It was hard for her to discuss—she was still feeling emotional about her mother's passing and the conversation brought back painful memories.

As time went on, she shared more stories about her mom with me. One in particular was quite disturbing.

My friend's mother had her own phone, and she and her daughter would talk with each other frequently throughout the day. On a few occasions, my friend's mother would fall asleep during their conversation. Her hand would fall on the bed with the phone line still open. Obviously, no one who came into the room was aware that someone could be listening on the other end of the open phone line. On more than one occasion, my friend heard one of the nurse's aides come into the room, remark that nothing had been eaten from the tray that had been placed on her mother's bed table, and proceed to remove it.

During those times, she never heard anyone attempt to wake her mother to encourage her to eat or try to feed her. Then, in subsequent visits to the facility, her mother would tell my friend that she was hungry because she hadn't eaten (either breakfast or lunch). When my friend would go to the nurse's station to report that her mother said she was hungry because she hadn't eaten, she was told she must be confused because she had been served whatever the previous meal had been. Of course, because my friend lived several states away and wasn't able to be there all the time, she could not dispute what she was told. However, from what she heard during those times when her mother had fallen asleep during their conversations, she believed that she hadn't eaten. Over time her mother began to deteriorate. She lost weight and became weaker until she eventually passed away.

What a gut-wrenching story, but unfortunately not unfamiliar. But that's not all there is to this story.

During the summer of 2018, my friend finally got around to the painful task of cleaning out her mother's apartment. She spent hours each day cleaning, painting, organizing, and wading through boxes of paraphernalia. She knew I was working on this book, and one day I received a text from her with an October 28, 1978, newspaper clipping from the *New Haven Register* her mother had saved all those years. It was a picture of my friend's beautiful mother as a young woman, presenting the award to the recipient, Grace Lenox Flight. My friend's mother was none other than Margaret Maunder.

Here was a woman who recognized the importance of improved quality of care for elder citizens by presenting an award to a nursing home administrator who also recognized that same need. All of these years later, she herself died in a nursing home, seemingly the recipient of substandard care.

While this predated the Nursing Home Reform Act, despite that landmark reform, the standards for care in nursing homes has not changed significantly. To this day many people continue to fear placement in a skilled nursing home facility.

Our aging parents, this country's elder citizens, live in a variety of settings in our society. Those who are able live independently, either in their own homes or in retirement communities. At some point, they may be able to remain in their homes but require assistance. Other individuals may enter assisted living facilities. In the event a person experiences physical or cognitive decline, he or she may require an increased amount of supervision or care. Eventually many may find themselves needing to move to a skilled nursing facility as they continue life's journey. This in no way should be considered a final destination, but rather a simple change in living environment that allows them to live a life with purpose and provides them with dignified and respectful treatment and quality of care.

The continual changing landscape of healthcare in the United States has created confusion and anxiety among those of us who are in the position of seeking care options for our loved ones, for friends and family members who are responsible for loved ones already residing in care facilities, or for those among us who are already living in care facilities. According to current reports, approximately 1.5 million individuals currently reside in nursing homes. Though there is little talk in our society about the aging process, we need to take a hard look at our attitudes toward our aging population, especially as the numbers continue to increase. Morningstar, the investment research firm, projects that by 2050, 15 million Americans will have high long-term care needs. There are substantial costs associated with the number of conditions an individual of advanced years might experience as well as with the end-of-life cycle itself. It is incumbent upon us as individuals, and society in general, to begin the conversation.

The cost of long-term care in the United States was estimated at $225 billion in 2015.[1] However, the quality of care our aging population is receiving does not appear to be equal to the amount of money being spent.

Our elder citizens deserve respect for the lives they have lived, but sadly oftentimes they are being mistreated. Many owners of skilled nursing-care facilities are getting extraordinarily wealthy, while those who live in these facilities are often neglected, mistreated, and even abused. It appears that the mindset of many of these owners is to provide the least that is required while gaining the most. I do not condemn owners for wanting to profit from their business. However, while these owners are in the "taking care of people business," too often, that does not seem to be their priority.

That is the unfortunate state of eldercare in America. In order to be the best advocate for an elder person—your mother, father, husband, wife, grandmother, grandfather, sister, brother, beloved aunt or uncle, or even a close friend—it is vital to take a hard look at how the elderly are being treated in these facilities. Indeed, the use of the word *facility* connotes exactly what these places have become: cold, stark, institutional settings, akin to a hospital-like environment. However, the term *nursing home* is better suited for what the situation is meant to be. These places are meant to be a person's living environment, a person's home, a place where they have to live for a variety of reasons as they continue their life's journey. As such, these "nursing homes" should provide a comforting living environment with the proper care needed to accommodate an individual's physical, mental, or functional limitations.

Investor-Operated, For-Profit Mega Corporate Facilities

Many skilled nursing facilities are operated by investor owned, for-profit mega corporations that own multiple facilities. They are hugely profitable (and this is almost an understatement). In 2014, of the 15,640 nursing homes in the United States, almost 11,000 were for-profit.

But if they are making so much money, why are conditions in many of these facilities so deplorable?

The problem of bad or even abusive care has not significantly changed in decades. Issues involved in investor-owned, for-profit healthcare corporations were reported by the Institute of Medicine based on a 1986 study entitled "The Changing Structure of the Nursing Home Industry and the Impact of Ownership on Quality, Cost, and Access."[2] The article not only examined the for-profit structure for hospitals but also the issues related to nursing homes that have been occurring since the 1970s. The results were astounding. Nursing facilities under for-profit corporations, as well as those that were part of a chain of ownership, spent fewer dollars on direct patient care, which of course resulted in reduced quality of care. The findings from additional studies throughout the years have been consistent with that study.

An analysis of the ten largest for-profit nursing-home chains for the years between 2003 and 2008 was undertaken in 2011. It compared for-profit ownership with not-for-profit. The findings were consistent with previous reports. Researchers found that across the board, for-profit facilities had:

- The lowest staffing levels
- The highest number of deficiencies identified by public regulatory agencies
- The highest number of deficiencies causing harm or jeopardy to a resident. (A nursing home deficiency occurs when a nursing home does not meet a particular requirement for a standard of care as set forth by Federal guidelines during a nursing home survey.)

The Government Accountability Office issued a report in 2010 that studied what is known as special-focus facilities. The program to study these facilities was created in 1998 as part of President Clinton's Nursing Home Initiative. The purpose was to identify nursing homes across the country that were providing the worst care and require them to undergo more frequent oversight through the state survey process. Thus, the Centers for Medicare and Medicaid Services (CMS) identified the poorest-performing facilities across the country and issued the following findings:

1. These facilities are more likely to be part of a chain and for-profit compared to other facilities.
2. They have fewer registered nurses per resident per day.
3. They are ranked lower on the CMS' five-star rating system.[3]

The Government Accountability Office issued another report in 2011 that focused on facilities purchased by the top-ten private-equity firms between 2004 and 2007 and found the following:

1. They had more total deficiencies than not-for-profit facilities.

2. They reported lower total nurse-to-patient staff ratios.
3. They showed capital-related cost increases and higher profit margins compared to other facilities.[4]

One can easily conclude that in general the type of ownership of a particular facility has implications for the quality of care being delivered to its patients and residents. What I find particularly interesting is that many of these "chains" include the word *care* in the company name; however, it appears that the primary focus of that care is directed toward the profit that can be extracted rather than providing the individual with the quality of care they deserve.

The Public's Right to Know

The Affordable Care Act addressed the seriousness of this issue by including a provision requiring full disclosure and transparency of the details of a nursing home's facility ownership to the Centers for Medicare and Medicaid Services (CMS) and for that information to be available to the public. When armed with knowledge of a particular facility's ownership, families would have a better chance of making more informed choices about where to place their loved ones. In addition, they would be able to investigate the reputation of that ownership, which could provide some knowledge and expectancy about the care that patient or resident would receive. However, oftentimes the complicated structure of nursing home ownership is mired in a web that is difficult to understand. An individual facility, or one that is part of a nursing home chain, may be structured for ownership in a variety of ways. These may include: for-profit corporations, not-for-profit corporations, limited liability companies, general partnerships, limited partnerships, or limited liability partnerships.

The question remains: despite the information available regarding for-profit ownership and its impact on care, why has this type of ownership been allowed to skyrocket? In the area of the East Coast where I have worked, over the past few years almost every not-for-profit facility or those that were privately owned have been bought out by a handful of these corporations. I know of one company that, because it's no longer able to purchase facilities in New York State, has recently bought a dozen facilities in a south-central state. A major investor in that company also has a stake in ownership in facilities in three other states in another area of the country.

What does this mean? First, restrictions should be put into place that would disallow the owner or owners of a facility that has been known to have significant deficiencies related to its standard of care from crossing state lines to purchase other facilities. This enormous problem can only be addressed by legislation.

Second, the proliferation of these companies across the country has serious implications for the ever-growing issue of the care of our nation's elder citizens. It is incumbent upon our nation's policy makers to devise reimbursement systems mandating that the dollars are spent on providing a level of care that is commensurate with decency and respect for our elders and removes the loopholes that allow owners huge profit margins.

The Nursing Home Reform Act

There have been some attempts to fix this very broken system. The Federal Nursing Home Reform Act of 1987 is widely considered the first major revision of the federal standards and practices for nursing home care since 1965, when both Medicare and Medicaid were created.

This legislation effectively changed the landscape for legal ramifications and expectations for individuals residing in nursing homes. It specifically stated:

Long-term care facilities wanting Medicare or Medicaid funding are to provide services so that each resident can attain and maintain his/her highest practicable physical, mental, and psychosocial well-being.[5]

It also created an ombudsman program—essentially a means for residents and families to voice complaints about any infringement of their care or their overall well-being to an impartial proprietor of sorts who would advocate on their behalf.[6]

The Omnibus Budget Reconciliation Act of 1987 (OBRA '87), often referred to as the Nursing Home Reform Act, outlined the basic tenets for nursing home care. They are as follows:

- Emphasis on a resident's quality of life as well as quality of care
- New expectations that each resident's ability to walk, bathe, and perform other activities of daily living (ADLs) will be maintained or improved with obvious consideration given to medical reasons
- A resident-assessment process leading to development of an individualized care plan
- Rights to remain in the nursing home except in instances of nonpayment, dangerous resident behaviors, or significant changes in medical condition
- New opportunities for potential and current residents with mental retardation or mental illnesses to receive services both inside and outside of the nursing home
- A right to safely maintain or bank personal funds with the nursing home
- Rights to return to the nursing home after a hospital stay or an overnight visit with family and friends
- The right to choose a personal physician and access medical records
- The right to organize and participate in a resident or family council
- The right to be free of unnecessary and inappropriate physical and chemical restraints

- Uniform certification standards for Medicare and Medicaid homes
- Facilities prohibited from turning to family members to pay for Medicare and Medicaid services
- New remedies to be applied to certified nursing homes that fail to meet minimum federal standards

The intention behind these regulations conjures up images of what could, and should, be provided to our elder citizens at the highest possible level. It is indeed unfortunate that the reality has not met our highest ideals, but rather has served as the backbone of an industry that has sought to capitalize from it.

This pattern must be stopped. The information in this book is meant to shed light on how the system is currently functioning, which is the backdrop of the landscape that must be changed. The alternative models presented in this book show that there is a better way, and hopefully encourage us that "we can do better."

It's Time for a Change

Skilled nursing care facilities are meant to be "taking care of people," but too often they are *not* taking adequate care of people but rather taking care to ensure that *their* bottom line is continually growing.

The way we care for this segment of our population reveals much about our society and our underlying values. The assurance that every individual deserves the highest quality of life as he or she continues through life's journey is one that each of us wants for ourselves. We should replace the phrase "dying with dignity" with "living with dignity to our final day." This is our basic human right.

We are all responsible to be part of this discussion, for as we age, we all will eventually be part of this population. As Stanislaw Jerzy Lec said, "No snowflake in an avalanche ever feels responsible." The funding, staff development and training, research, and continued oversight of our long-term-care facilities will determine the quality of our future, and raising public awareness about this is why I wrote this book. Each one of us should be willing to speak out on this issue, not only for our loved ones, but for *ourselves*. Unless we work in this field or have experience with a loved one in long-term care, it is all too easy for us to close our eyes to these issues. "Out of sight, out of mind" is not merely a euphemism. Our elder citizens *are* essentially locked away out of sight and therefore, we are not mindful of what is happening. The purpose of this book is to open our eyes so we as a people can see what is happening and do something about it.

In the words of Madeline Albright in an interview regarding her latest book, "If you see something, say something. Now I'm saying, do something."

We are the consumers here. The skilled nursing care facility industry is regulated by the federal government, but the system is broken and it is up to us to demand change—both for our loved ones and eventually for ourselves.

TWO

ELDERCARE IN AMERICA— A MORAL DILEMMA

"Of all the forms of inequality, injustice in health care is the most shocking and inhuman."
MARTIN LUTHER KING JR.[7]

SEE ME[8]

What do you see, nurses, what do you see?
Are you thinking, when you look at me—
A crabby old woman, not very wise,
Uncertain of habit, with far-away eyes,
Who dribbles her food and makes no reply,
When you say in a loud voice—
"I do wish you'd try."

Who seems not to notice the things that you do,
And forever is losing a stocking or shoe,
Who is unresisting or not, let you do as you will,
With bathing and feeding, the long day to fill.
Is that what you're thinking, is that what you see?
Then open your eyes, nurse, you're looking at ME . . .
I'll tell you who I am, as I sit here so still;
As I rise at your bidding, and I eat at your will.

OVERDUE

I'm a small child of ten with a father and mother,
Brothers and sisters, who love one another,
A young girl of sixteen with wings on her feet,
Dreaming that soon now a lover she'll meet;
A bride soon at twenty—my heart gives a leap,
Remembering the vows that I promised to keep;
At twenty-five now I have young of my own,
Who needs me to build a secure, happy home;
A woman of thirty, my young now grow fast,
Bound to each other with ties that should last;
At forty, my young sons have grown and are gone,
But my man's beside me to see I don't mourn;
At fifty-one more babies play 'round my knee,
Again we know children, my loved one and me.

Dark days are upon me, my husband is dead,
I look at the future, I shudder with dread,
For my young are all rearing young of their own.
And I think of the years and the loves that I've known;
I'm an old woman now and nature is cruel—
'Tis her jest to make old age look like a fool.

The body is crumbled, grace and vigor depart,
There is now a stone where once I had a heart,
But inside this old carcass a young girl still dwells,
And now and again my battered heart swells.

I remember the joys, I remember the pain,
And I'm loving and living life over again,
I think of the years, all too few—gone too fast,
And accept the stark fact that nothing can last—
So open your eyes, nurses, open and see,

Not a crabby old woman, look closer, nurses—
See ME!

Was it always like this?
Is it like this everywhere?

Our attitude toward and treatment of the elderly, sick, frail, and infirm is just as much a stain on our nation's social conscience as is the history of racial injustice. Major national platforms focus on the care of our children. The issues of drug addiction, obesity, mental health, and AIDS have been catapulted to a national conversation. Loud and persistent voices have most recently elevated the MeToo Movement, Black Lives Matter, and Gun Violence to that conversation. However, there is little or no mention of changing our attitude toward eldercare and the devaluation of life in advancing years which, according to a 2018 study by the Yale School of Public Health, contributes to the cost of health care for older adults to the tune of $68 billion.[9] This as an issue of human rights. As human beings we are entitled to live our lives with the highest level of purpose we can achieve, taking into consideration our physical abilities, limitations, and mental capacity.

An examination of the way other cultures treat their elderly compared to American culture reveals a huge disparity stemming from deeply rooted attitudes and beliefs—not only in philosophy but in use of terminology. Word choices shape our attitudes; consider these common phrases often used to talk about our aging population:

- They are in their declining years.
- He's over the hill.
- She's in her old age.

Wikipedia defines *old age* as: "nearing or surpassing the life expectancy of human beings and thus the end of the life cycle."[10] In some way we've created a brand, an image in people's mind, of what older people are like, how they behave, what they are able to do, and how much they can still contribute. Yet there are people who act "old" at forty, and ninety-year-olds who act in a way much younger than their chronological age. We've all heard the rare individual who says, "I'm ninety years young." This is not a contradiction in terms, not something to be laughed at, but an attitude to be admired. I'm sure I am not alone when I say I have known individuals in their eighties and nineties who are alert, spry, and have a sharpness of wit second to none. According to a theory known as stereotype embodiment, as a child if you think older adults are weak and frail, that will most likely become a self-fulfilling prophecy as you yourself age. A person can unconsciously internalize this idea across the span of their lifetime.

Thus, attitudes toward aging are essentially a social stigma that are artificially manufactured as a result of societal and social thought.

The U.S. Attitude Toward the Elderly

To American youth and many young adults, older people are an intrusion, a nuisance, an annoyance, and a burden. In our fast-paced, immediate-gratification society, where we have no time for ourselves—let alone others—there is no place for the amount of time, effort, and patience needed to care for our aging citizens.

A young man at a conference shared with me a philosophy he heard from a gentleman friend from Ghana:

> It is said that when a young child dies in America, we mourn it as a tragedy for the loss of the potential and an unfulfilled life; but when an "old" person dies, though mourned, we consider that they have lived a full life and reached their potential. However, death is

viewed from a different perspective in Ghana. When a young child dies, the child's passing, while tragic, represents an unfulfilled life, and therefore the loss of what has not yet been revealed is not a tragic as the loss of an old person. When an elderly person dies, it is considered that a library is lost.

While there may be more TV commercials depicting care, medication, and consideration for parents with Alzheimer's, dementia, or other ailments associated with older citizens, they are still few and far between. We would like to think it is so much easier these days to find a place for senior adults to stay and assume they will be cared for in a respectful, decent, and dignified manner. But is this the realty? Are we deluding ourselves into believing that our loved ones are being treated respectfully, decently, and with dignity because we cannot bear the burden if this is not the case and because we are not willing to assume the responsibility? I postulate that the answer to that is, unfortunately, yes.

It's Not Only a U.S. Issue

While it is not integral to our culture—as it is with some others—to respect or value older people, taking care of an aging population is statistically becoming a worldwide problem.

In 2000 there were 600 million people in the world aged sixty and over. This number is expected to increase to 1.2 billion by 2025 and 2 billion by 2050. Today about two-thirds of all older people are living in the developing world, and by 2025 it is predicted to be 75 percent. In the developing world, the eighty-plus population, considered as the "very old," is the fastest growing population. According to a U.S. Census Bureau's 2017 report, by 2030 all baby boomers will be older than sixty-five; essentially one in every five residents will be retirement age. At the time of this book, that is only twelve years away.

By 2035, the number of people sixty-five and older will outnumber those that are less than eighteen years old—78 million people aged sixty-five as compared to 76.7 million younger than eighteen.[11] It's seems so far away for most people. They don't think about it, and they can't even envision it. It's like something in the distant future, but for a substantial part of the population, we are talking about ourselves in the near future. We save for retirement, but do we think about how we will be treated when we get there? The time is here, the time is now, for the elder citizens today—and for ourselves tomorrow.

For instance, the elderly population in Japan is growing exponentially. Statistics report that by the year 2020, 7.2 percent of the Japanese population will be eighty years old or older.[12] Supplies necessary for older citizens are selling in greater numbers than those for babies, and pension funds are expected to dwindle or dry up entirely.

Jeremy Hunt, the secretary of the National Health Service (NHS) in Great Britain, gave a speech entitled "Elderly Treatment 'National Shame.'" He said that England should be ashamed of how it treats the elderly and that, according to the Campaign to End Loneliness, eight hundred thousand chronically lonely elderly people existed in English society. Family members who do not visit the elderly leave them feeling isolated, and people should examine how they treat their own parents and grandparents.[13]

He said, "If we are to tackle the challenge of an aging society, we must learn from this and restore and reinvigorate the social contract between generations."[14] Hunt also stated that health care has to be more human and patient-centered and less system and bureaucracy centered.

We certainly see this in the United States. It is counterintuitive that the nursing-home industry has become a business rather than a patient-care model. But the patient-care model is one that should be reconsidered entirely. Patient care, as it is today, consists of a medical-based model; this misplaces the "care" in the hands of the medical community. The business aspect of the medical model is at cross purposes with much of what the elder citizen requires because it revolves around profit and loss, not human compassion and dignity.

Certainly, there must be a medical management component when caring for elder citizens who may suffer from a variety of ailments, and this has given rise to the field of geriatric medicine. However, long-term care facilities also should be places where the individual's rights and desires and quality of life are given priority, resulting in an atmosphere that addresses their psychosocial needs.

Other Cultures and Their Attitude Toward the Elderly

When we examine the traditions of different cultures and their treatment and care of older persons, we quickly see the effect of deeply rooted philosophical, religious, and ethical beliefs. I present a few as examples.

China

In China, treatment of the elderly has as a core principle the concept of filial piety, or *xiao*, where respect for parents, elders, and ancestors is considered a fundamental virtue. It can best be described as one based on age or rank, regardless of family ties or affiliations. If one looks up the Western definition of the words *filial* and *piety* one would find that *filial* means "being or due from a son or daughter"; the word *piety* means "dutiful and devout." Therefore, if one was to stick to the Western definition, that relationship would be restricted to one's own family.

Confucianism also outlines the way family members should treat one another and interact, but the philosophy actually goes deeper than that. The Chinese use a character to express filial piety that is comprised of a top portion that depicts an old man with a young man underneath, supporting him. It can be viewed by typing "filial piety character" into the search bar at seniorsaloud.com.

The notion of filial piety exists not only between an elder and younger person in the family unit, but also extends far beyond to include any elder and younger person in society as a whole. This is a powerful symbol. The depth to which *xiao* is ingrained in Chinese culture and psyche is best seen by the fact that it extends to one's ancestors and can be described as an ancestral relationship whereby even ancestral worship is valued.

It's hard for Westerners to fully understand this concept. Many of us tell stories of our parents and grandparents, as much as we remember. I lost my father forty-eight years ago, and with the passage of time, I no longer think of him on a daily basis. But there often are stories or situations that creep into my consciousness and I find myself referring to them in conversation. That is how I continue to honor his memory—that is how we all honor the memory of our loved ones who have passed. But reverence and respect for our ancestral line is on another level altogether.

As increasing numbers of people respond to advertisements for companies that help trace ancestry, a possible shift is beginning to emerge. However, this pertains more to the individual's interest in finding out about his or her roots and does not extend to influencing the culture on the importance of the ancestral relationship.

Integral to this relationship in the Chinese culture, however, are attributes of respect, reverence, duty and responsibility, tolerance and patience, provision and welfare, kindness, love and affection, and loyalty.

In China, the family does not exist as an independent unit but is the foundation of society. In essence, one's existence and identity are integral to the family and the ancestors from which the family originates; they are interdependent. In the Chinese culture, you are nothing without your family, which is why neglect of one's elders is considered shameful and a blemish on the family name. Furthermore, the *xiao* relationship does not only apply to how one treats elders but extends to how one addresses them. In essence, filial piety is a moral code of conduct and is considered fundamental to achieving familial, societal, and social harmony.

In actuality *xiao* did not emanate from the teachings of Confucius alone. Its roots can be found in Taoism and Buddhism, and the influences of Taoism and Buddhism are crucial to understanding the full extent of the tenet. According to Taoist beliefs, *xiao* must flow naturally and be freely expressed—not forced, compelled, or contrived in any way. Compelling *xiao* can result in intense resentment and be entirely counterproductive. In accordance with Buddhist philosophy, the virtue of *xiao* is an act of gratitude and repayment of sorts for the parent's boundless, limitless kindness, caring, and love.

The guiding principle of what the Chinese call the "Filial Piety Sutra" is that a parent's lifetime of care is considered so difficult to repay that "it can never be compensated even if one were to carry one's parents on the shoulder without putting them down for a hundred or a thousand years."[15] The "Filial Piety Sutra" outlines ten ways in which the mother especially bestows loving-kindness upon the child.

The "Filial Piety Sutra"
- Providing protection and care while the child is in the womb
- Bearing suffering during the birth
- Forgetting all the pain once the child has been born
- Eating the bitter herself and saving the sweet for the child
- Keeping the child dry even if it means she has to stay in the wet
- Suckling the child at her breast, nourishing, and bringing up the child
- Ensuring that the child is clean and healthy
- Always thinking of the child when he or she is away from home
- Deep care and devotion
- Ultimate pity (i.e., worry) and sympathy

When Confucius lived, the tenets of *xiao* and filial piety became mandatory in fourteenth-century society as a means of achieving social harmony. Those times were turbulent, troubled and war-torn; therefore, filial piety is identified with Confucius.

In modern times China is facing challenges to filial piety that are akin to situations in our own country. With the advent of younger people moving from remote areas to the city to find work and working long hours, children are finding it difficult to take time off or use their resources to visit or care for family members. In addition, the Chinese restriction of one child per family has put a tremendous strain on the sole offspring, who must in some cases provide for both parents and grandparents.

Because of this awareness of an ever-increasing older population, the Chinese government made an unprecedented ruling in 2015 to increase the family allowance of children from one to two. As it is around the world, where advances in medicine are increasing life expectancy, the result is an increase in the aging population for which nursing homes are emerging as an option for elderly care. This is compounded by the trend in China, as in other countries such as Japan and India, where young people want privacy and a home of their own.

Small living spaces in the cities are not conducive to the option of extended family members living under one roof, and older family members who have lived their life in remote areas do not want to move to the city. The result is elderly citizens without financial means or emotional support and no way to meet physical needs as they become increasingly frail.

Up to now there has not been a provision for societal eldercare in China. However, because the concept of filial piety is so ingrained in the Chinese culture and way of life, the government has passed an Elderly Rights Law warning "never to neglect or snub elderly people" and requiring children to visit their parents often, regardless of distance—though there is no definition of "often."[16] In addition, adult children are responsible for providing financial, emotional, and physical support for their parents. (I have seen these ideas embraced in many families from many different cultures throughout my years working in skilled nursing facilities; however, it is certainly not the "norm" and not one embraced by the culture at large here in the U.S.) In China, on another level altogether, parents are even entitled to sue their children if not given adequate financial support.

The Chinese government has tried to require businesses to allow time off for children to visit their parents. There are potential penalties for not complying with the law that range from fines to jail time. This is a direct contradiction to the basic Taoist principles that *xiao* cannot be forced or compelled, and there are reports of tremendous resentment resulting in neglect and physical and emotional abuse. Because of these trends, nursing homes are emerging as acceptable alternatives for elderly care in China.

Korea

The influence of the Confucian principle *xiao* also extends to Korea, where respect and value for older citizens is considered a fundamental virtue. Reaching sixty years old is considered a rite of passage into old age and is worthy of celebration. Similarly passage into the seventies is marked by significant birthday celebrations. As parents age, it is considered honorable and an adult child's duty to care for parents. Placing parents in a retirement home could earn the adult child the label of being an uncaring or bad son or daughter.

The essence of Confucianism followed in Korea can be seen in the following: "Few of those who are filial sons and respectful brothers will show disrespect to superiors, and there has never been a man who is respectful to superiors and yet creates disorder."[17] *The Huffington Post*, in an article on cultures that respect elders, relayed the message, "A superior man is devoted to the fundamental. When the root is firmly established, the moral law will grow. Filial piety and brotherly respect are the root of humanity."[18]

India

It is common practice in the Indian culture to find joint or multigenerational units living together under one roof. The elders become heads of the household, and adult children provide support and cater to the elders' needs. The elders in turn play a major role in raising the grandchildren. Elders are placed in high regard: they are sought out for advice on a range of societal, personal, and even financial issues. There is considerable stigma associated with abrogating responsibility by sending elder family members to any type of old-age or living situation outside the home.

Philippines

The act of showing respect to the elder population in Philippines is similar to other Asian countries. This is conveyed both by gestures as well as by the words they use before the person's name. Any younger person addressing an older person is expected to use a specific word (*po* or *opo*) before the person's name to show respect; to do otherwise is considered to be an act of rudeness. This reminds me of how I was raised as a child. One could not address any adult by their first name, but, always by Mr., Miss, or Mrs. Is it possible that by allowing our children to address adults by their first names, we have lost a sense of respect?

The word *po* is used to show respect when responding to an older person who has beckoned to you and is also used in conversation when addressing someone older. The word *ate* is generally used for older sisters or cousins and is said in front of a person's name if she is female. *Kuya* (meaning brother) is used for a male. Without exception, I have seen this used amongst my Filipino and Filipina colleagues.

There is also a gesture used to show respect to elders known as *mano po* or "bless." Upon greeting an elder, the younger person takes the outside of the hand of the elder and places it against his or her own forehead. This action could be considered akin to a priest who places a hand on the forehead as a way of blessing. Therefore, the use of *mano* (the hand) and *po* (bless) is a way for the young to show respect for their elders.

Native Americans

Native American spirituality centers around honor, love, and respect—for the creator, all living things, the earth, and each other. It is the

Native American tradition that elders are valued for their knowledge and wisdom and are expected to pass these things down to the younger members of the family.

The widely held belief is that elders hold the answers, keep the culture alive, and deserve the utmost respect. This attitude is summed up in a quote by White Feather, a Navajo medicine man: "Native American isn't blood; it is what is in the heart. The love for the land. The respect for it, those who inhabit it; and the respect and acknowledgment of the spirits and the elders. This is what it is to be Indian."[20]

There are over five hundred federally recognized Native American tribal communities, each with unique attitudes, traditions, and customs. The prevailing point of view is that elders should be able to remain at home and in their community as they advance in years, known as "aging in place." It is considered to be a continuation of ancient customs of extended and lifelong care for family but also the result of the many years of social isolation and discrimination experienced by Native Americans relegated to living on reservations their entire lives.[21]

An excerpt from the *Inter-Tribal Times*, published in 1994 on the Native American code of ethics, says:

> Treat every person from the tiniest child to the oldest elder with respect at all times. Special respect should be given to elders, parents, teachers, and community leaders. No person should be made to feel "put down" by you; avoid hurting other hearts as you would avoid a deadly poison.[22]

Greece

In most Mediterranean cultures, several generations often live under one roof, and there are words to address elders that connote extreme respect and reverence. This is especially true in Greece. In Greek culture the concept of *philotimo* involves generosity, hospitality, and respect for others—especially elders. Furthermore, the culture values seniority:

elders are thought to possess wisdom that is an accumulation of years of experience, which is to be respected. This philosophy is epitomized in this quote from BeNeca Ward: "We were taught to respect everyone, especially those who were older and wiser than we were, from whom we could learn."[23]

The Greek word for honor, *hubris*, is associated with renowned literary works *The Iliad* and *The Odyssey*. It dates as far back as the late eighth or seventh century BC, leading to the conclusion that since ancient times honor has been an important consideration in Greek culture. That honor now extends to modern Greek society, where family honor is considered to be a cornerstone that can be destroyed by the action of one family member. However, recent crises in the Greek economy have severely impacted caring for its elder citizens. The severe financial measures to maintain functioning society as a whole found pensions for senior citizens slashed by almost 40 percent, and privately owned care facilities experienced harsh tax increases that were passed on as price increases to residents and their families.

The programs available for seniors in Greece are mainly adult daycare centers and in-home programs, as the country does not have state-funded, long-term care centers. However, funds for these programs have been affected by significant financial cuts commensurate with the economic crisis, as well as reported mismanagement of funds.

Two organizations are trying to bridge the gap in this area. The Lifeline Program, which began in 2011, delivers bags and boxes of food to approximately nine hundred elderly people in Athens on a monthly basis. It has introduced a twenty-four-hour-per-day, seven-day-per-week, pager-alert system whereby an elderly person at home can contact someone in the event of an emergency. It also operates a national helpline for those elderly citizens who are neglected or abused or who are experiencing medical or family issues. A program established in 2005, known as 50+, promotes elder citizen rights and provides incentives for them to be active in society.

There may be further challenges to come for the elder citizens in Greece if the financial climate results in deeper pension cuts and shrinking social-program funding that may all but disappear.[24] The situation in present-day Greek society is a disheartening and stark contrast to the philosophy of ancient Greece, where it was considered a sacred duty of the children to look after the elderly. It's a sad commentary indeed that when societal finances are strapped, support for the citizens that contributed to that society are often scrapped. And this is no different to what occurs in the United States.

France

There has been an interesting development in France regarding eldercare that is unrelated to an underlying filial-piety-type philosophy. In 2004 an Elderly Rights Law passed, due largely to statistical information reporting that the highest rate of suicide was among "pensioners" (sixty-two deaths per week). Adding impetus to the legislation was a horrific situation in which 15,000 elderly people died as a result of a crippling heatwave. Their bodies, in a staggering number of cases, were unclaimed for weeks because their families were on annual holiday.

Article 207 of the French Civil Code requires children to honor and respect their parents, pay them an allowance, and provide or fund a home for them; repercussions for not doing so can result in fines or imprisonment. The law stipulates that it is a crime if children do not keep abreast of their parents' medical conditions if they live alone and requires them to intervene if parents become ill. According to a parliamentary report, "It is not acceptable that children exonerate themselves from all responsibility for their aged parents."[25]

As in the United States, in France there is a fascination—almost an idolization—of youth. Dr. Renee Arnaud-Castigliioni, head of the psychiatric service for the elderly at Marseilles Hospital, says that society "overvalues the image of youth at the expense of the elderly."[26] In the United States, the youth culture is highly valued along with independence, individualism, and self-reliance. This, along with the Protestant work ethic (i.e., if you're no longer working, your societal value is significantly diminished), impacts attitudes toward our older citizens. What younger people fail to realize when they are looking askance at an elder person is that they are looking, hopefully, at their future selves: a concept that is understandably hard to grasp. Who among us ever thought we would actually reach this age? I think there is a fallacy in thinking that if we do not think about it, it will not happen to us. Or conversely, if we do think about it, we automatically become an elder person. It is far too easy, to look away, to deny its existence.

From a technological viewpoint, to many people the older generation has also lost its usefulness. Contemporary literacy and access afford us the ability to use search engines to find information. What young people miss is that in procuring information in this way, what is lost is the flavor and the context of rich family stories and traditions. This is what other cultures value as the wisdom associated with knowledge. The information gleaned from a search engine cannot give advice. It creates a false conception that information and personal knowledge result in better decisions than the wisdom that comes with years of experience, which only an older person can provide. As Jared Diamond so beautifully states, "The repositories of knowledge are the memories of the old people."[27]

It's Time for a Change

The General Assembly of the United Nations established what it termed an Open-Ended Working Group on Ageing[27] in December 2010 for the purpose of protecting the human rights of older persons with the results undertaken as part of the world human rights convention. It held its ninth session July 23–26, 2018.

Being "elderly" is a generalized term that creates stereotypical thinking not applicable to everyone who falls in an age range. There are people who are alert, vital, and active in the later stages of life—some who continue to work well into their seventies and eighties. Appropriate intervention is more than a function of chronological age.

I prefer using terms such as "elder or older citizens" or "aging parents." By using the term "aging parents," we acknowledge that these people are our parents—directly and indirectly, individually and collectively. Without them we wouldn't be here. Without us as parents, the next generation would also not be here. As elder citizens, we acknowledge that they have been active, contributing members of our society—a far more dignified description. Dignified terminology is usually followed by a sense of respect that encourages dignified action or treatment. One flows naturally from the other.

We *must* do better in this regard. As the conversation on national health care addresses much-needed health care for all of our citizens, there also needs to be a national conversation about meeting the needs of our elder citizens in a more dignified and respectful manner. This conversation must be without consideration for the accumulation of astronomical profits by a few who, along with the rest of us, will become sick, old, and infirm one day and will want better care for themselves and their families.

John McCain said, "We are better than this." He couldn't have been more correct in our attitudes toward our elders. Change begins within. It is imperative that every person take a hard look at how he or she views the elder person. We should have the utmost respect for our aging parents, and we should demand that they be treated as we would like ourselves to be treated—with kindness, respect, and decency.

PART TWO

THE "NUTS AND BOLTS"—
HOW THE SYSTEM WORKS

THREE

THE STATE SURVEY PROCESS

The Department of Health Survey and the Nurses Association Appreciation Dinner

The director of the Rehabilitation Department told me that the administrator invited her to attend a holiday Nurses Association Appreciation Dinner; he had bought several tables. She went to the dinner, but did not see the Administrator there and wondered why. When she told me the head of that particular Nurse Association Appreciation Dinner was also the head of the local Department of Health Survey Team, it made sense. That's why this facility had a five-star rating on the Nursing Home Compare website, when it didn't deserve more than three stars at best, and that was probably being generous. This was the same facility that I'll describe later in the book as having horrible food; small, rundown, grungy-looking dining rooms; and residents eating in hallways. I explained to my friend that of course the administrator could not show his face at the dinner; that would be too obvious. But the fact that the company bought several tables at the dinner did not go unnoticed when it came time for the facility's annual survey.

This is an example of the extent people are willing to go in order to continue making money while providing as little as possible to those entrusted to their care. In this case, the Department of Health Survey

Team was complicit with the owners by allowing them to continue in that fashion. While this is the only example I'm aware of, I wonder if any similar situations have happened in other facilities.

THE SHORT FAT GUY AND THE MILLION-DOLLAR BUDGET SAVINGS

He was literally a short, fat guy. He stood approximately 5 feet 8 inches tall and weighed around 350 lbs. His shape looked like a barrel—excessively rotund around the middle. His dress was always the same: a white shirt and a pair of black trousers held up by a black belt. His clothes were ill-fitting, the shirt sloppily tucked into the trousers and always seeming to be creeping out of them as he walked. His overly large midsection protruded over his belt like a potbellied stove. Surprisingly, though, he moved quickly for his size. He exuded an energy that loomed large wherever he went, not only because of his excessive weight, the rapid pace of his walk and size of his steps, but also because of his persona. He was foreign born with an intensity and aggressiveness that filled up the entire area wherever he went. He spoke in a deep, booming voice that was almost deafening. He also had an aura of invincibility, mainly because of his relationship with the facility administrator—his best friend with whom he was practically joined at the hip. They had worked together closely for years.

His position at the facility was director of food service. He was responsible for overseeing food purchasing and budgeting, meal preparation, kitchen personnel, kitchen staff scheduling, and serving appropriate diets required by all patients and residents based on doctors' recommendations.

To call this "short fat guy" a braggart was an understatement. He openly and repeatedly bragged to many staff members about how he had saved the owners a million dollars in the year he had been working at the facility. In addition, he was functioning as food service director for two of the other three facilities under the umbrella of this group's ownership. He also talked about saving at least one of the other buildings a half a million dollars in food service costs. He touted this as the reason they recruited him to work for them.

It is not surprising that residents of the main facility where the "short, fat guy" worked frequently complained that both the taste and quality of the food had deteriorated since he arrived. They complained that they no longer received fresh fruit, the menu choices were limited, there was little variation from day to day and week to week, and the menu did not reflect seasonal changes. I questioned him about this last one several times. He shrugged it off, indicating he would get to it when the new computer system became active. To this day I don't understand what one had to do with the other. Ultimately, when I left the facility mid-summer, I saw little change in the menu choices even though the computer system had already gone "live." It was apparent that his bragging about the financial savings to the ownership took precedence over the resident's satisfaction and well-being.

When I arrived at this particular facility, I observed a dietary issue that was impacting the residents' quality of life as well as their safety and well-being. Certain of the residents required a modified consistency diet due to dysphagia, a swallowing problem, and many of them referred to the food they received as "dog food." Instead of food that was supposed to be served in the form of a chopped consistency, these residents were receiving food that was more of a ground consistency. Indeed, it did resemble dog food.

I worked closely with the "short fat guy"—he was one of the greatest allies I ever had in a food service director up to that point. He said he recognized that the facility was "missing" a consistency and was "all-in" in working with me to develop it. We worked together tirelessly. We developed lists of foods that could be served in a more recognizable and pleasing fashion. We educated the cooks on food preparation and those who served the food on which foods were appropriate to be served on each consistency. As a result, many of the residents were now able to have an upgrade in the consistency of the food they ate. They were extremely happy and appreciative. This was all accomplished in approximately six weeks, really record time. Suddenly I realized that the frenzied pace was related to the impending Department of Health's annual survey. At the time, I was elated that this "project" seemed important to the administration. They couldn't bestow enough accolades regarding what I brought to the facility and how that improved the quality of life for the residents. The takeaway was that the residents would then speak favorably about their satisfaction with the food and its consistency during the New Resident-Centered Survey. There were obvious glitches along the way, which is to be expected when a new process is implemented in such a short period of time. I conducted in-services, or short classes, to educate all levels of the nursing and rehabilitation staff. Things were going fairly well up until and shortly following the survey.

When the facility passed the survey without a single mention of a deficiency, everyone was understandably ecstatic. But shortly thereafter, things began to slide. Those responsible for serving the food became sloppy, and the nursing staff—primarily certified nursing assistants—who went up to the serving station to request the food for the residents eating in the spacious main dining room also became careless. Residents began receiving the wrong consistencies, placing them at risk for serious consequences, mainly choking. Both the servers in the kitchen and the CNAs were repeatedly educated about the importance of providing appropriate food consistencies and the risks and consequences of not doing so. The "short fat guy" repeatedly pointed the finger at nursing, and nursing repeatedly pointed the finger at the servers in the kitchen. However, as I always emphasized in my educational sessions, the last person who places the food in front of the resident is ultimately responsible for ensuring that the appropriate consistency is served. That person is what I call the "last line of defense" for that individual. It is their responsibility to read the resident's meal ticket, which is in essence a doctor's order, and ensure that the food on the plate is in accordance with what is supposed to be served.

Shortly thereafter, with the arrival of the summer months, the facility had problems with the air conditioning system, resulting in scorchingly hot temperatures. This went on for weeks as the outside temperature hovered in the high nineties. The air was stifling—hot and humid. Both staff and residents could hardly breathe; it literally felt like a sauna. The feeble attempts at importing portable air conditioning units were ineffective. As a result, the residents could no longer eat in the main dining room.

Therefore, all the meals were served to residents on their respective units. The errors that occurred were beyond egregious. On each of the seven floors of the facility, for each meal, there errors occurred repeatedly concerning both solid and liquid consistencies. It was brought to the attention of the nursing staff each time, but it also highlighted the extent of the incompetence of the servers in the kitchen who were responsible for assembling the trays, reading the meal ticket, and providing the appropriate foods and food consistencies, both solids and liquids.

A meeting was called to address these serious issues. The interdisciplinary meeting was attended by the administrator, the director of nurses, the assistant director of nurses, the dietitian, the medical director, the food service director (the "short fat guy"), the two speech pathologists (one of them being me), and the director of the rehabilitation department. Suggestions and recommendations were bantered about, and finally a few were agreed upon. However, at the conclusion of the meeting, the medical director opined that, despite the efforts of the team, she did not think the situation would change. It was discouraging, disappointing, and alarming to hear a medical director state matter-of-factly, in a cool and calm voice, that the situation with serving residents the wrong food and consistency would not be remedied with the recommended solutions that came out of this meeting. She expressed no alarm, no insistence that the situation had to change. It made me wonder about her commitment to the well-being and safety of the residents.

What was even more concerning to me was that "the short fat guy" with whom I worked so closely to develop the new chopped consistency diet, stated unequivocally that he "intended to get rid of that consistency as soon as I walked out the door, even though he knew it was better for the residents." (Indeed, I had resigned and was scheduled to leave the facility in a few weeks.) The reason he gave was that it was too much trouble to go back and forth with nursing about the foods that should or should not be on the trays. I told him that I was extremely disappointed and it seemed totally disingenuous. The hard work to create a new diet consistency was akin to a sham for the purposes of the Department of Health annual survey.

The "short fat guy" did not seem to care. After all, he accomplished his two main objectives: 1) to save the owners a million dollars in food costs, and 2) to have the residents report feeling satisfied with the food during their interviews with the Department of Health surveyors. Resident satisfaction, quality of life, and overall well-being no longer concerned him.

This brings me back to another description of the "short fat guy." He presented himself as being devoutly religious. However, this entire way of behaving seems totally counterintuitive to that premise, doesn't it?

Why am I telling this story?

This facility consistently passed its annual survey, often without even the most minor deficiency. In addition, it had a five-star rating on the Nursing Home Compare website.

It is also important for people to know that problems with diet consistencies are serious issues.

A person who receives the wrong solid or liquid consistency can develop aspiration pneumonia, choke, or even die. After all, the only thing that belongs in our lungs is air. Anything else entering our lungs is known as aspiration. Many of us have experienced the feeling of food heading into our wind pipe. The cough reflex is our body's way of expelling whatever substance is "headed the wrong way." Sometimes it might even be the smallest amount of our own saliva. The intense coughing as we attempt to expel whatever food or liquid particle is attempting to enter our lungs as we gasp for air can be painful and scary.

I shared the above story so family members might become vigilant about ensuring that their loved ones receive the appropriate food consistency. They should insist that any errors in consistency that occur be immediately reported to them and accurately and thoroughly documented in their loved one's medical record.

In the June 24, 2016, *USA Today* "Money" section, the headline below the fold read: "Wall Street Banks Ace Fed's Severe Stress Test."[28] As encouraging as this headline sounds, one need only to turn the page and see the headline at the top of the left-hand page to find the irony: "Bank of America Fined $430M for Cash Misuse."[29]

This disparity caught my attention because it relates to the annual state survey process for skilled nursing facilities and the star-rating system. In addition to the example above, I personally know of many other facilities listed as five-star that function in a way that makes me question how that could be possible. They pass their annual state survey every year, some without even a single mention of an infraction. While the notion of a star-rating system intuitively seems like it would be a measure of conveying quality of care and services to the public consumers of health care, it doesn't necessarily function the way it was originally intended. The desire for a facility to obtain a high-star rating is often based on circumstances having nothing to do with the quality of care that is actually being provided.

My personal experience is in New York State, but around the country on blogs, websites, and in newspapers, there are many reports of nursing homes that passed their respective state surveys only to have later been found with egregious deficiencies and poor quality of care. There is also a website updated monthly (see appendix) that adds facilities to the federal watch list, naming those with the most egregious deficiencies and those that provide the worst care.

These types of discrepancies moved the State of Illinois—on January 1, 2016—to become the fifth state to pass a law allowing cameras to be placed in patients' rooms as a means of chronicling care and ensuring there is no mistreatment or abuse.[30]

While the nursing-home industry is heavily regulated by both federal and state regulatory bodies, the Government Accountability Office acknowledges that the annual inspections by the department of health in each state "tend to understate the number of serious nursing home problems that present danger to residents."[31] The article says that a report issued in September 2008 indicated that 94 percent of nursing homes received citations for deficiencies in the health or safety categories in 2007 and that in 17 percent of the facilities those deficiencies were in the category of "actual harm or immediate jeopardy to patients."[32] In actuality, between 1997 and 2010 there were more than twenty reports issued by the Government Accountability Office that cited substandard care in many nursing homes, understated (serious) deficiencies by state surveyors during annual surveys, unenforced sanctions for resident harm, and both ineffective and inconsistent oversight by the federal government, all of which obviously were not protecting the health, safety, and welfare of nursing-home residents.[33]

The ProPublica website reported an egregious situation related to poor care at a particular New York facility. Despite the record of "repeat fines, violations, and complaints for deficient care in recent years,"[34] the founders of the organization with that facility under its umbrella had been allowed to continue buying nursing homes, placing the organization at the top of the list of that state's largest networks of nursing-home ownership. Prior to buying additional facilities, proposed buyers are supposed to undergo a state character-and-competence review to ensure that the other health-care facilities owned by the prospective buyer have a record of high-quality care.[35] This is an example of how flawed the system really is.

How can this happen when there are state oversight agencies

conducting annual reviews and charged with identifying and reporting those issues? The agency charged with the final decision in these situations is the Public Health and Health Planning Council, which consists of appointed individuals—many of whom have direct ties to the health care industry.

It is within the council's jurisdiction and authority to urge prospective nursing home buyers to improve quality of care within their existing homes, but an examination by ProPublica into many of these transactions in recent years shows that this is not happening. Furthermore, the council is supposed to have the Department of Health's character-and-competence recommendation prior to making the decision. A departmental report of one of the principal owners of that company and his partners found that the facilities offered a "substantially consistent high level of care," which is the necessary requirement to receive approval. The company received this commendation despite the fact that twenty fines had been paid to the federal government in fifteen of the facilities under that company's ownership since 2013. There was no mention of the infractions or the payment of these fines in the commendation.

The owners and their relatives and/or associates also applied for ownership in many facilities in 2014. To date they reportedly have ownership shares in over thirty facilities inside and outside of New York State. In over a dozen cases, the Department of Health reported that there were "no repeat violations," yet this organization's nursing home facilities were cited on multiple occasions for repeated serious deficiencies.[36]

ProPublica reviewed many nursing home deals besides those of this particular company and found that a green light was given despite the rules firmly stating that deals shall not be approved when facilities have repeat violations involving substandard or poor care placing residents at risk. The interpretation that is often applied to give the stamp of approval to these deals is that approval can be granted if the violation or deficiency is not identical or if the facility addressed the deficiency in a timely fashion.

"Advocates for nursing home patients say that instead of a backstop, New York's approval process has become a rubber stamp. The law establishes mechanisms for at least a moderate review of an applicant's character and competence," said Richard Mollot, director of the LTCCC in New York. "The failure to provide complete information on a provider's past performance fundamentally undermines the review process.[37]

In a recent report, Richard Mollot states that the Department of Health, which is a regulatory agency charged with nursing-home oversight in New York State, has "one of the nation's lowest rates of citing nursing home operators for deficiencies in care."[38]

The Centers for Medicare and Medicaid Services is a federal regulatory body that sets forth the parameters for the survey process. The process is carried out by the department of health, which is the overseeing body for nursing home facilities in each state, and its findings are subsequently reported to Centers for Medicare and Medicaid Services. In order for skilled nursing facilities to receive Medicare and Medicaid reimbursement, they must be found to be in compliance with that agency's guidelines. In New York State, the Department of Health oversees nursing homes through its Division of Nursing Homes and Intermediate Care Facilities for Individuals with Intellectual Disabilities Surveillance. This division is the agency that acts on behalf of the federal government's Centers for Medicare and Medicaid Services, which monitors quality of care in nursing home facilities.

Surveys are conducted annually, within a period of up to fifteen months from the previous survey. They are unannounced, and surveyors may arrive at a building at any time. However, it should be noted that most facilities carefully follow the whereabouts of survey teams in their area; therefore, the facility can usually gauge when the team is due to arrive. Though I have seen survey teams arrive in the very early morning hours (six to seven o'clock) and sometimes on a Friday, they more typically arrive on a Monday or Tuesday and conclude their visit by the end of that week.

In September 2016, in a surprise move, the Centers for Medicare and Medicaid Services announced a new nursing home survey process which was a response to years of outcry by systemic advocacy groups that the process, and the system in general, was heavily based on regulatory information and review of papers and computers, but did little to look at or consider the individual. Thus, it touted the new process as being more person-centered. The new process was scheduled to be introduced in three phases over a three-year period. Phase 1 (November 2016) included very minor changes to the existing requirements; Phase 2, slated to become effective November 28, 2017 (to include all Phase 1 requirements); and finally, Phase 3 which will include the above 2 phases and become effective November 28, 2019. After pressure from owners, the Centers for Medicare and Medicaid Services put a hold on some of the changes that were to go into effect in November 2017. Once again, the desires of owners superseded the needs and well-being of our elder citizens.

It is this author's opinion that the public should be aware of the areas being examined in order to fully understand the survey results. Therefore, I've attempted to explain the information in a way that the reader does not get lost in the detail.

Furthermore, if families already have loved ones in a facility, they should be aware of what the survey is looking at specifically so they can speak out about the reliability of the results compared to their actual day-to-day experiences. I think that most residents and their families believe they are at the mercy of the ownership and can do or say little to effect a change. But in actuality, residents and their families are the customers, and as customers, it is up to us to demand better service.

Though we are on the precipice of the anticipated advances that the new regulations and the new survey process will have on the safety, quality of care, and lives of our nation's long-term care facility residents, it appears that the lobbying efforts of providers continue to take precedence. As with other questions in our society today, this should be a moral issue, not one based on politics. On October 11, 2017, 120 members of the House of Representatives signed a letter presented to the Centers for Medicare and Medicaid Services for the purpose of reevaluating the requirements, citing the burden they represent to providers. What will it take for this vicious cycle to end? When will a higher ground of morality finally prevail?

As previous outlined, Centers for Medicare and Medicaid Services stipulated a three-year timetable to phase in these changes, from 2016–2019. Despite years of preparation, some have requested that the phase-in enforcement period be suspended entirely pending a finalized version of a new rule, while others call for delaying Phases 2 and 3, the phases with the most critical and crucial changes. In response, the Centers for Medicare and Medicaid Services has agreed to a moratorium on selected Phase 2 requirements. In the meantime, our nation's nursing home residents become older, sicker, increasingly frail, and vulnerable.

The Centers on Medicare and Medicaid Services is already considering reneging on some of the regulations: reporting of abuse and neglect, the Quality Assurance and Performance Improvement process, and discharge notices to long-term care ombudsman. In addition, they have reopened comments on any other areas of the requirements that would result in "reducing the burden" and serve as cost-saving measures to long-term care facilities (i.e., the ownership). By doing so they have essentially opened the door to modifying or eliminating many more of the current regulations stipulated in the October 2016 ruling. This process will allow representatives of nonprofit and mainly for-profit facilities to once again exert their influence and continue their indefatigable efforts to pursue financial gain over quality care for the almost one and a half million nursing home residents.[39]

As recently as May 2018, the issue of rolling back nursing home reforms remained an ongoing concern. As a result, seventeen attorneys general of the United States signed a letter that was submitted to the Centers for Medicare and Medicaid Services. The following are excerpts from that letter.[40]

> We write this letter to express our concern and to alert the Centers for Medicare & Medicaid Services (CMS) about the substantial and foreseeable detriment of CMS' actions to delay enforcement of protections for Medicare and Medicaid beneficiaries who receive care in skilled nursing facilities (SNFs). The recent CMS guidance significantly decreases the protections in SNFs by rolling back reforms to improve the safety and well-being of nursing home residents. If allowed to proceed, recent regulatory changes will not only threaten the mental and physical security of some of the most vulnerable residents of our states, but also potentially create additional challenges for MFCU investigation and prosecution of grievances, violations, and crimes occurring in SNFs. We therefore urge you not to lower the level of regulatory oversight. . . .
>
> The proposed regulatory roll-back comes at a time when the U.S. population is aging and in need of quality care in safe facilities.

It goes on to cite familiar statistics: that by 2060 the population over the age of sixty-five will double and more of those individuals will need to seek out skilled nursing facility to meet their healthcare needs. Furthermore, one in three individuals will find themselves at some point in their lives in a nursing home environment. It further states that of the 1.4 million people in nursing homes in 2015, over 60 percent of them experienced some type of cognitive impairment.

> Ensuring that this expanding vulnerable population receives quality care will require significant resources, including those for reporting abuse and for enforcement activity against bad actors.

On May 4, 2017, as part of a proposed rule published in the Federal Register, CMS requested feedback on "Possible Burden Reduction in the Long-Term Care Requirements." Since then, despite the fact that no formal rulemaking has taken place, CMS has issued memoranda to decrease the amounts of Civil Money Penalties levied against non-compliant SNFs and to delay the enforcement of the 2016 long-term care regulatory reform. These actions weaken existing protections for SNF residents and roll back critical reforms.

We as State Attorneys General recognize that Civil Money Penalties are an essential tool for regulators to ensure SNF compliance and guarantee better performance in the future. Consequently, weakening or delaying their application hampers our ability to both punish bad actors and ensure improvement, thereby putting beneficiaries' lives at risk. For instance, the July 7, 2017 guidance instructs CMS Regional Offices to impose lower per-instance penalties rather than per-day penalties for past violations. These changes decrease the dollar amount and frequency of penalties that—though rare and low in amount—nonetheless did help safeguard Medicare and Medicaid beneficiaries. The threat of penalties is a deterrent to SNFs engaging in abusive behavior. Eroding even these penalties enables unscrupulous SNFs to provide substandard care and receive minimal penalties, if these lapses are even brought to light.

The 2016 long-term care regulatory reform included provisions to increase infection control; improve training for SNF staff; and provide protections against abuse, neglect, and exploitation of Medicare and Medicaid beneficiaries. The components of these regulations were scheduled to take effect in three phases, the second of which was due to take effect on November 28, 2017, before CMS acted to delay implementation of certain penalties by 18 months. Enforcement of these reforms keeps SNF residents safe and healthy. They should not be put off or discarded.

The letter went on the discuss the poor quality of care that individuals receive in skilled nursing facilities. It cited the fact that in 2016, 34.3 percent of all skilled nursing facilities were cited for violations of quality of care and 20.1 percent were found to have actual harm or jeopardy to a resident and that of the over 15,000 facilities in the U.S., only 6.5 percent were found to be deficiency free during their annual state surveys. The letter cited a statistic from California where 170 citations were issued to skilled nursing facilities in just the first four months of 2018, and some of those included citations for patient abuse.

The Office of the Inspector General issued a report on August 24, 2017 which stated that "CMS has inadequate procedures to ensure proper identification and reporting of incidents of abuse or neglect at SNFs." The report went on to say:

> Approximately 22 percent of Medicare beneficiaries experienced adverse events—including infections, pressure ulcers, and medication-induced bleeding—during their SNF stays. Nearly 70 percent of these adverse events could have been avoided if the SNF had provided better care, and over half of residents who were harmed required hospital care. The number of violations at SNFs demonstrates that beneficiaries are in need of more protection, not less.
>
> To remove important protections for SNF patients amounts to a devaluation of human wellbeing. Further, these actions to arbitrarily delay or capriciously remove protections are an abuse of federal law. Rolling back regulatory reform and decreasing penalties for non-compliance will result in less governmental oversight of behavior in the long-term care industry. . . .
>
> We urge you to reconsider this ongoing regulatory rollback. Protecting the health and security of some of our most defenseless people is a special charge we as States, together with CMS, must uphold.

Why wasn't this letter signed by the Attorneys General of every one of the fifty states? Is it because of political affiliation? Is it because the lobbying efforts by owners are too pronounced in the other thirty-six states?

Furthermore, why was it necessary for this letter to be written? While the necessary regulatory bodies recognized the importance for enacting legislation to improve the quality of life and safety of our loved ones in skilled nursing facilities, it only proves that they remain vulnerable to lobbying efforts that would negate the very same legislation they felt the need to enact. A sad fact indeed.

Admittedly, some progress has been made on at least one of these issues. A November 2018 *Kaiser Health News* article reported that the federal government has now ordered more surprise inspections on weekends to "catch" facilities reported to have been understaffed on Saturdays and Sundays. The short staffing was able to be identified through reported payroll records. Some of these facilities not only are understaffed on the weekends, but also operate without a registered nurse on the premises. Federal law requires that each facility have an RN on duty at least eight hours a day, seven days a week. The *Kaiser Health News* report found 11 percent fewer nurses and 8 percent fewer nurse aides respectively available on weekends to provide direct care.[41]

However, another *Kaiser Health News* report[42] indicates that owners of more than half of the nursing homes in California have requested to be exempt from the state's new regulation regarding staffing which passed as part of the state's budget bill. The regulation requires facilities to have more staff available who are directly responsible for patient care. The owners' objection was based on the fact that they thought was too burdensome for them to comply and were unable to hire sufficient staff. The California Department of Public Health is expected to issue an announcement in their January 2019 reporting if any nursing homes that filed to be exempt would actually have their request granted.

Staffing requirements for nursing homes are long overdue: advocates believe the regulation does not go far enough. It is appalling to think that any consideration would be given to granting an exemption from a staffing regulation when understaffing has been the hallmark of many nursing homes and substandard care. The literature substantiates that increased staffing creates more favorable outcomes, improved care, reduced falls, and fewer pressure sores. California should be applauded for being one of a few states that has set a staffing requirement, as most other states in the country prefer to abide by the original federal guidelines which stipulates that facilities only have to provide "sufficient staffing," a phrase open to interpretation, too often to the detriment of nursing home residents. Some California nursing home officials have reported that it is difficult to find staff to meet the needs; however, with salaries kept at low levels, and reduced staff that creates burdensomely high workloads, this is to be expected. The article points out that some of the nursing homes seeking exemption from the ruling are the same ones that have been cited for patient harm resulting from inadequate staffing. One of the owners who falls into this category owns one in fourteen nursing home beds in the state of California and has been faced with "numerous federal and state probes of understaffing and quality problems at his homes."[43]

I reiterate that this issue should be separate from political affiliation. The care of our elder citizens is a moral issue—a dignity issue—*a human rights issue*. It's an issue of respect and dignity—two of the "pillars" set forth in the nursing home reform act (OBRA) of 1987. These are our parents, individually and collectively. As it has been said, we are to treat others as we would ourselves. For those of us who live to become elder citizens, we are advocating for the treatment we ourselves will receive in the future.[44]

Furthermore, the seriousness and lengths to which many among us go to preserve life at its very incipient stages, involving a few cells in a woman's body, should be an exact measure to which all of us cry out against the injustice of how we treat the elderly, frail, and infirm among us. These should not be cast away because they are no longer able to adequately care or speak for themselves.

Survey Results and Deficiencies

Federal deficiencies in skilled nursing facilities are rated in terms of scope and severity; in other words, the widespread and flagrant nature of infractions. An A-level deficiency is considered to be the minimal level, while the L-level is the most severe. Examples of minimal deficiencies where there is no potential or actual harm for residents include things like an omission note on an individual plan of care, a document without a signature, or a missing therapy note. The survey team shares these findings, determines the reason for the deficiency, and allows the facility to make the appropriate corrections to avoid such mishaps in the future.

The final department of health survey report should always be readily available and in a place where it can be easily viewed in every facility, such as the hallway or dining room. Any person, whether a visitor, family member or resident, has the right to view the report. In addition, the phone number for anonymous reporting of concerns or infractions should be listed throughout the facility. Though it is rarely put into practice, the policy is, "If you see something, say something." Under the new survey process, everyone in the facility is a mandated reporter. Anyone who is witness to, or has knowledge of, abuse of any kind within the facility is obliged to inform local law enforcement.

It appears that the state survey process as an oversight for nursing homes is sufficiently encompassing to identify potential sources of inadequate or poor quality of care that would negatively impact residents. Therefore, since facilities are annually audited by state surveying bodies—technically every fifteen months—one would not expect to see a facility with extensive egregious failures. It should be rare to see deficiencies escalate to the immediate jeopardy level or see care so substandard that facilities are placed on a federal watch list.

So why is it that these things are not as uncommon as we would expect? An ABC News article entitled "Report Finds That Lack of Enforcement Allowed for Neglect at State Nursing Homes" published on July 26, 2016, may provide some insight. Pennsylvania Auditor General Eugene DePasquale essentially found that the Department of Health was remiss in its documentation, adherence to standard protocols, and enforcement, which resulted in neglect and allowed unsanitary conditions in nursing homes to "slip through the cracks."

"What this tells me is the Department of Health was not looking," DePasquale said during a press conference. "And when you don't look, there's no way to discover problems." In the same article, he goes on to say that nursing homes that "failed to meet state standards were often not cited during Department of Health Inspections."[45]

The question is a moral one: why are the regulatory agencies charged with overseeing nursing homes not looking? Will a new survey process be the solution to impact the much-needed change in the care of our elder citizens residing in nursing homes and skilled nursing facilities?

The facility I mentioned at the beginning of this chapter participated in the new survey process. And yet the team did not carry out one of the very first mandated tasks after they arrive in a building: observation of a meal service in a dining area.

- Why did they not complete that mandated task?

- How was the fact that they didn't observe the meal service documented in their report?

- Was it because they were somehow "tipped off" that it was a chaotic situation (as indeed it was), leaving it open to serious errors in food consistencies being served to residents with swallowing problems? Such a situation could certainly result in the facility being cited for a deficiency.

• Was it because the ownership purchased several tables at the nurses' association dinner chaired by a survey team leader?

• Will this new survey process significantly impact the care currently provided in facilities? Or will the changes, while possibly rooted in research and good intention, wind up to be nothing more than window dressing on an already flawed system?

FOUR

THE STAR RATING SYSTEM

The Good, the Bad, and the Ugly:
How Some Facilities Get Their Star Rating

One of my colleagues contacted me asking if I would come build a speech program in a nursing home where she had become the director of rehabilitation. I was familiar with the company that owned this facility as I had worked in two other buildings under their umbrella several years prior. Knowing the owners and how they ran the other facilities, I was somewhat reluctant but finally acquiesced.

I walked into the building for my scheduled prehire meeting with the administrator of the contract agency responsible for the company's hiring. There was a small reception area with a dusty artificial plant and an outdated table that also had a thin layer of dust. Completing the scene was an inexpensive lamp with a crooked lampshade and an electric cord dangling from the table as it ran along the wall to the outlet. It was vastly different from many of the more modern-looking facilities I was used to seeing.

The security guard asked me who I was there to see, but when I told him, he barely recognized the name and had no idea where he was or how he could be reached. It felt awkward and struck me as very unprofessional. There was no chair, so I was forced into the balancing act of struggling to hold my purse, the folder with my professional papers which I would present during my meeting with Mr. S., and my cell phone which I was using to try and call him. I finally opted for texting him. After about ten minutes that seemed like an eternity, he finally arrived. We went through a maze of stairs and hallways until we finally came to another building where his office was located.

Mr. S. was a man in his late thirties or early forties. He had an engaging personality and expressed some of the most forward-thinking ideas I had ever heard from someone affiliated with the ownership of a nursing home. He acknowledged that Certified Nurse Aides were some of the most valuable but unappreciated workers in a facility and said that a strong recreation department offering a wide range of activities was an important ingredient for keeping residents engaged. He believed this could be an enormous benefit for the individual resident to counteract the boredom that often was a root cause for some resident's so-called "acting out" behavior.

He went on to say that speech therapy was almost a department unto itself, and therefore, they did not impose the same productivity requirements on the speech/language pathologist as they did with therapists from other disciplines. I especially liked the fact that this family-owned business seemed content with the four nursing homes under their umbrella and were not looking to become major players in the corporate world of nursing home ownership, as was the case with most of the companies with which I worked in recent years.

I left the meeting thinking that perhaps a younger generation was bringing a new approach to the facilities and this may be a good move for me. From the conversation with Mr. S., I was expecting to work in a facility with great emphasis on resident happiness and well-being. We agreed to touch base by phone in the next few days. Indeed, within a week we agreed on a date when I would begin working at one of their buildings.

When I arrived at the facility a few weeks later, as I walked through that dreary, dated reception area, I was now wondering why, with such a forward-thinking administration, the area looked as it did. Yes, the facility was in a crowded, urban area with a lower socioeconomic profile, but I still thought it should still look a bit more presentable and professional.

I was led into the conference room for the first morning report meeting to be introduced to the staff. This meeting is usually attended by all department heads to review the facility census (the number of occupied beds), individual resident concerns, incidents, facility concerns, important facility news, and so on. Mr. S. made an appearance to ensure I was properly introduced and welcomed appropriately. He seemed proud to have hired someone with my level of experience.

I began work as I usually do—having meetings with the director of the rehabilitation department (the colleague who asked me to join her there), the dietitian, and director of the food service. The rehabilitation department director told me she was sure I would identify important issues that needed addressing almost immediately.

My first order of business was to make meal rounds. This involves visiting the various dining rooms (one on each of the six floors) during meal service. In this facility, the meals were prepared in the kitchen, and the completed trays were then sent up to each unit to be distributed to the appropriate resident by the nursing staff.

The first-floor dining room was the main dining room, located on the same floor as the dreary, dated reception area. Residents on this floor could leave their rooms and enjoying eating in a large, bright room with many windows at one end. On this day in early December, the sun was shining brightly through the windows, giving the room an almost warm glow in sharp contrast to the cold weather outside. However, I noticed that some of the venetian blinds were broken. This small but important detail seemed in contrast to the rest of the room, and I made a mental note of it as I proceeded to the upper floors.

The second-floor dining room, although much smaller, was nicely decorated. This floor was set aside for patients who were there for short-term rehabilitation. The furnishings, room décor, and bathrooms on this floor were more "upscale"—a stark contrast to the dated reception area.

From there I continued to the remaining four upper floors. What I found was appalling: small, dreary, faded beige-colored dining rooms with dirty, broken venetian blinds and an isolated, crooked old picture here and there on the walls. Many of the brown, fake wooden tables were crooked, unstable, and had small pieces broken off at the corners, exposing the cheap synthetic material underneath. The sharp edges were rough and could easily cause a skin tear or bruise on the skin of an older, infirm person. There were not enough stools for the staff who had to assist the patients with eating and the ones that were there were so old that the vinyl tops were ripped and cracked. Besides being unsightly the sharp edges could easily scratch anyone who attempted to sit on them.

The conditions were deplorable, and my eyes welled up with tears. It was so sad to see the surroundings that sick, frail, and infirm residents were forced to experience while eating their meals. How could anyone consider this an acceptable dining experience? How could anyone sitting in these surroundings even want to eat? What did this say about the administration's attitude toward the residents? Far different from my impression after my initial meeting with Mr. S.

Some of the dining rooms were not large enough to fit all the residents, especially since some of the more impaired residents had to be seated in larger reclining geri-chairs.[46] On one particular floor, I observed residents eating in the hallway. This obviously raises a red flag about dignity. I found out later that for purposes of the Department of Health survey, a nurse manager was coerced into writing on the care plans of certain residents that eating in the hallway was their choice. I don't know how those statements were considered acceptable for survey purposes, as several of these residents were extremely impaired, confused, and unable to respond or express their needs and wants. Certainly, they would not have been able to indicate they wanted to eat in the hallway. Thus, this became an exercise to satisfy paper requirements, but had little to do with actual resident care. It's a sad fact that it was a situation that was in plain sight but was obviously overlooked during the state survey process. One could not think it was anything other than intentional.

As horrible as the appearance of these dining rooms was, the food was worse. I heard residents say it looked like "s--t" on a plate, or like dog food. The smell was horrendous, almost putrid. The sandwiches had virtually nothing in them; they looked like two pieces of bread pasted together. Most of the residents on most of the floors did not eat the meal.

As I did my rounds from one dining room to another, I also found that many patients on the units were not positioned properly for feeding, whether sitting in the dining room or in their respective rooms. I attempted to educate, correct, and assist the staff in proper and safe positioning for eating, but the information was not received well. The impression I got was that the staff felt this was an imposition and that, because they were short-staffed, they did not have time to address the idea of positioning residents properly during meals. Many of the patients were being served their meals, or being fed, lying almost flat. I pointed out to the staff that they themselves would probably not eat in that position; nor would they allow any one of their children or loved ones to eat in that way as it could cause choking.

I returned to the rehabilitation department and reported my findings to the director. She told me that is exactly what she too had observed and, like me, felt so sad for the residents. She arranged for us to meet with the administrator.

Over the next two months, the rehabilitation director and I repeatedly spoke with the administrator about the deplorable food and overall conditions of the dining rooms. I suggested painting the dining rooms a brighter or more appealing color, replacing the venetian blinds, and possibly hanging some colorful window treatments. Considering the small size of the four dining rooms in question, the cost would probably not amount to much more than a thousand dollars. I also continually brought up the situation with the stools and suggested ordering three more per dining room.

The food was a more serious concern. I began taking pictures of the plates of food served on the units. Not only did they look terrible, food consistency for those with swallowing difficulties was also a serious issue. I repeatedly suggested the formation of a committee responsible for "dining rounds," the purpose of which was to observe the problems with the food being served. The group could consist of people from various departments: social service, recreation, occupational therapy, speech therapy, the rehabilitation director, the director of nursing, the assistant director of nursing, the food service director, and the dietitian. On a particular day, two to three members of the group could visit various dining rooms once or twice weekly and report their findings to the remainder of the group in order to identify problems and come up with solutions. Ultimately, the administrator, director of nursing, and director of rehabilitation visited the dining rooms during meals on a couple of occasions, but the committee was never formed.

After two months, the only change that was implemented was the purchase of stools for the various dining rooms. No other changes were instituted. I even suggested that the administrator contact two of my colleagues at other facilities where they served relatively good food. Each of them said they'd agree to visit the facility at no charge, as a professional courtesy, to give suggestions to the food service director about improving the taste and quality of the food being served to the residents. The administrator never contacted either of them, despite me asking him about it repeatedly. Finally, after several months, the administrator told me it wouldn't do any good because the food service director wouldn't implement the suggestions. I did not understand. After all, he was the boss. Wasn't he concerned that just about every resident complained about the food? Residents who had sufficient funds were constantly ordering food from the outside. Others who did not have the means or ability to order out were losing weight. The director of nursing also suggested that the Food Service Director visit a few other facilities to get ideas about improving the quality of the food being served. She did not follow through on those suggestions either.

I felt so horrible about not being able to make a change for the better that I attempted to resign twice. The administrator did not want to accept my resignation, and the second time I submitted a resignation letter, Mr. S. came to speak with me. He assured me he would somehow try to improve the situation. Because of my favorable impression with Mr. S. during our first meeting, he was able to convince me to stay.

As time went on, though, I became increasingly disheartened about the conditions for the residents in the facility. I was relentless in my complaints to the administration, imploring them to do something to improve the surroundings and the food, but my pleas fell on deaf ears. The only change I heard about was that they were planning to convert that spacious, bright dining room into a new and improved rehabilitation department. This would attract more Medicare-insured, short-term rehabilitation candidates for which the facility would receive a higher reimbursement rate. Once again, the focus for increased revenue supplanted the interest in improving the surroundings for the residents who lived in the facility on a long-term basis. There was hustle and bustle as architects and designers visited the facility to present their ideas. And then, if that wasn't bad enough, during this time I also found out the most incredulous information.

This was a FIVE-STAR facility!

How could that be?

The food and dining experiences alone were deplorable, and the staff seemed uncaring. Though elder citizens are out of sight, and essentially out of mind for society at large, these conditions were in plain sight. The job of the Department of Health state surveyors is to provide oversight to ensure that residents' dignity and well-being are integral to the care provided by the facility. Anyone visiting the facility could readily see this was not the case.

So how could this facility have received a five-star rating?

This facility was owned by the same company described at the beginning of the previous chapter in which the administration purchased several tables at the local nursing association dinner, the director of which was a state surveyor. While it is uncertain if this is the only reason the facility attained a five-star rating, in my mind, the possibility could certainly not be ruled out.

<hr />

Nursing Home Compare is a database that lists and ranks all licensed nursing home facilities throughout the country by assigning a star rating system (five stars being the best) in an effort to help consumers determine which facilities to choose for themselves and their loved ones. Facilities can be located by name, as well as by city and state. The website also includes information on ownership and whether a facility is for profit, not for profit, or government-owned and operated (see appendix for website address).

Facilities achieve their star ratings based on determinations in each of the following three categories:

1. Health Inspections Rating—This rating is based on the latest three years of the annual department of health surveys and is supposed to take into account information from both the standard on-site surveys and any other surveys that may have been conducted as a result of complaints. The most recent inspection report carries more weight than those from previous years. This is important information for anyone looking into a facility for placement.

2. Quality Measure Rating—The quality measure rating takes into account information from anywhere between eleven to sixteen physical and clinical measures in the facility that impact a resident's life. This does not include information about the how the facility utilizes antipsychotic medications for both long-term-care residents and short-term patients. The use of antipsychotic drugs is an important issue in skilled nursing facilities and one that people should understand and know about. It has been used far too widely as a way of restraining patients and attempting to make them more compliant. Furthermore, they are also used as a means of controlling behavior in light of reduced staffing. Changes to the guidelines have rattempted to reduce or restrict their use; however, overuse of these dangerous drugs persists.

3. Staffing Rating—Historically, staff rating information was based on information that was reported from the facility itself. Of course, a facility would report information that would cast them in the most favorable light and earn the most star ratings for that category. It took into account both registered nurse (RN) hours per resident, per day, and total staffing hours per resident, per day. Total staffing hours was determined by the number of licensed practical nurses (LPNs), licensed vocational nurses (LVNs), and Certified Nursing Assistants (CNAs). These numbers were looked at based on the levels of care needed by the residents of the facility or on a particular unit (e.g., sub-acute care, more clinically involved or complicated, or dementia unit).

The Affordable Care Act (Section 6106), recognizing that this was not an honest representation of what facilities were actually contributing to the detriment of the care provided, came up with what seemed to be a reasonable solution. Facilities are now required to electronically transmit payroll reports of regular, agency, and contract staff to their respective state. This system does not leave room for subjective interpretation or ambiguity.

The first mandatory reporting period began July 1, 2016, and it must be reported by the end of the forty-fifth day following each fiscal quarter. The system allows the data to be verified and, combined with census information from that facility, can be used to determine actual staffing levels as well as employee turnover and tenure, all of which impact the quality of care. This information can be published and made available to the public. The Centers for Medicare & Medicaid Services has created a system for reporting this information known as the Payroll-Based Journal (PBJ).[47] However, colleagues of mine recently told about me about a facility that passed its annual Department of Health survey without a single mention of a deficiency, when in fact, despite the new payroll reporting system, a significant number of caregivers were added at the time of the survey.

Facility star ratings can be found on the Nursing Home Compare website, which also contains a downloadable copy of the statement of deficiencies for any facility (whether it was the annual Department of Health survey or any other survey)—including the name of the nursing home, date it received the deficiency, tag number, scope and severity of the deficiency, and the current status and/or corrective action for the deficiency. Additionally, the report contains all penalties, including the number, amount, and payment details for any fine associated with the deficiencies that were imposed on a facility.

More detailed information on the star-rating system can be found in the *Five-Star Quality Rating System Technical Users' Guide*, which contains an in-depth description of the ratings, methodology, and calculations.[48]

A facility's staffing rates and ratios, citations, and quality-measure performance may be compared with both state and national averages. This is extremely important information for anyone who is looking into nursing home placement for themselves or a loved one. When choosing a skilled nursing facility, it is also always wise to make an on-site visit and be armed with a list of pertinent questions specific to your loved one's condition and needs or about the facility in general. (Suggestions for pertinent questions are listed in the appendix.)

In many instances, however, there is insufficient time to make an on-site visit. Hospitals may inform patients and/or families of an upcoming discharge without much notice, often placing them in the position of having to make a hasty decision under extreme pressure. In many cases the patient or family has never considered placement in a facility and therefore relies on information from either word of mouth or the Nursing Home Compare website, which may not be reliable. They also fall prey to the attractive glossy marketing brochures, professionally designed websites and smooth-talking admissions representatives.

Even more disheartening are the cases where an older, more compromised patient without family support or advocacy is unwittingly placed in a facility based on availability, marketing, or the hospital's relationship with that facility. (I actually knew of a marketing specialist from a facility owned by a large corporation who had a permanent office in a local hospital. In my mind, that situation certainly raises ethical questions.) The patient arrives in the facility not knowing where he or she is or how he or she got there; one can only imagine how disturbing that must feel. If the facility is one with substandard care practices, there can be even stronger physical and emotional implications for the patient.

Important Considerations

There are important caveats when considering the Nursing Home Compare star rating system as a guide for choosing a nursing home. First, one can easily see that the rating system and the survey results are interdependent. The star rating system, which is so reliant on survey results, is significantly problematic. There are numerous studies, newspapers articles, personal accounts, and blogs regarding the lack of identification or reporting of substandard nursing care—even to the extreme of serious abuse or neglect. Furthermore, the scope and extent of the deficiency are often underrated or in some cases not reported at all.

Second, as with staffing levels that were previously self-reported and based on a form the nursing home completed in preparation for its annual state survey, one can easily see that it is within the facility's best interest to shed the most favorable light on the care and attention that will be given to the resident or patient. After all, this is a business and the patients and residents are the customers. The goal of every business is to get more customers. This is why for many years the buzz word in nursing homes has been "customer service."

Quality measures are also self-reported and unsubstantiated. Thus, one can assume that the nursing home would be inclined to report this information to its advantage. As of 2015 the Center for Medicare and Medicaid Services began implementing improvements affecting the reporting of quality measures and has added antipsychotic drugging rates to the star rating in that category.

One example, as reported in the 2014 *New York Times* article entitled "Medicare Star Ratings Allow Nursing Homes to Game the System," reinforces the problem with the rating system—more specifically, the five-star rating.[49]

The article is about Ken Chandler who took his elderly mother to the Rosewood Nursing Home in 2011. The facility was a small, 110-bed facility with a five-star rating in a suburb of Sacramento, California. Rosewood was a picture of opulence and luxury and gave the impression it was deserving of the five-star rating.

As is the case with many for-profit nursing homes in recent years, the owners renovated the facility—especially the lobbies, rehabilitation units, and rehabilitation departments—to convey a luxury, high-end appeal. Rosewood's lobby, for example, resembled a luxury hotel with all the accoutrements—high ceilings, leather chairs, and serene paintings of pastoral landscapes. Ken Chandler and his wife were suitably impressed by the five-star rating and the hotel-like appearance.

Chandler was unaware that, despite Rosewood's five-star rating, it had been fined $100,000 in 2013 for the death of a woman in 2006 that resulted from an overdose of a powerful blood thinner medication. In addition, according to the California Advocates for Nursing Home Reform, from 2009 to 2013 there had been 102 complaints filed against Rosewood; some say the complaints actually numbered approximately 164. Rosewood had also been the subject of approximately a dozen lawsuits in recent years from patients and their families claiming substandard care.

Ken Chandler placed his mother in Rosewood after she had sustained a fall that resulted in a broken femur. Chandler's mother experienced several serious falls while she was a resident at Rosewood and died a few months later. Subsequently the family filed a lawsuit against the facility.

The article reported that the family felt misled by the rating system, which had played a significant role in their choice of Rosewood for their mother. Mrs. Chandler was quoted as saying, "You don't know where to look to get accurate information. I can go and find a preschool for my child better than I can find a skilled-nursing facility for my loved one."[50]

The *New York Times* article goes on to say that nursing homes, despite having a history of poor care, continue to receive high ratings—especially in areas such as staff and quality measures that are self-reported. "Of more than fifty nursing homes on a federal watch list for quality, nearly two-thirds hold four- or five-star ratings for their staff levels and quality statistics."[51]

The percentage of facilities that achieved a four- or five-star rating was 39 percent in 2009; in 2013 that number had risen to 52 percent. Some believe this was related to a transitional survey that was used, known as the Quality Indicator Survey. The drawback was that there were only a limited number of parameters that the surveyors were allowed to examine, and these were generated by a computer analysis of that facility. The computer-determined parameters were stringent, and the team was not permitted to look beyond them, notwithstanding an egregious noncompliance.

There are also agencies that track nursing home star ratings and work with facilities to help them bolster their ratings. The self-reporting of staffing ratios that helped determine the number of stars for that category was based on a form the nursing home completes in preparation for its annual state survey.

From personal experience in the over forty homes in which I have worked, I can attest to the fact that staff had been intentionally added near the time of the inspection. Workers throughout every facility have been aware of this and had complained of "working short" until it was time for state inspection. This practice had allowed the facility to complete paperwork reflecting higher staffing ratios in time for the survey. These false numbers were then reflected in the survey results and reported on the Nursing Home Compare website, thereby giving the false impression of adequate staffing ratios during the majority of the year. This was a way of duping the public. As with everything, staffing costs money. The goal of business is to minimize spending and maximize profits. It is uncertain if the full effect of the new payroll reporting will be reflected adequately in the star ratings and in the survey results, as evidenced by the example in the facility I mentioned earlier.

The same *New York Times* article quoted an excerpt of an e-mail that was included in a lawsuit filed that year against Medford Multicare Center, located on Long Island, by the New York attorney general. David Fielding, the nursing home's administrator, wrote about the state survey, saying that "the inspection period is so crucial" that it is like "our Super Bowl" and stating that following the state inspection, staff levels would drop. Fielding went on to write that "the staffing hours will be a little high for this week but will drop the following week."

Though the public relies on the Nursing Home Compare website and the star rating system to make the best choices possible to meet health-care needs, consumers are being misled. One may conclude that the rating system seems to be based on shielding ownership from the repercussions associated with noncompliance and substandard care rather than protecting residents entrusted to their care. Therefore, when looking to the star ratings, my advice is to view them with caution.

The purpose of the new "client-centered" survey is to obtain information about patient/resident satisfaction with the services they receive directly and whether those services fulfill their needs regarding overall well-being, quality of life and quality of care, dignity and respect, and freedom from unnecessary and inappropriate physical and chemical restraints. (Note: *chemical restraints* refers to the use of antipsychotic medications.) It will be interesting to see if the results of interviews with residents, many of whom are dissatisfied with the services they receive, the staff that administers those services, and the overall environment in which those services are delivered will impact survey results and, ultimately, the facility star ratings.

The Centers for Medicare and Medicaid Services will provide additional information regarding this matter on the Nursing Home Compare website in the future. In addition, in response to cries for improved transparency of nursing home ownership, Nursing Home Compare has begun to reflect this information when reporting facility deficiencies and poor-quality care. However, there is a greater need for transparency of deficiencies as it relates to nursing home ownership chains.

Information on the new survey process is contained in the *Revision to the State Operations Manual* Appendix PP for Phase 2 which also includes a revised F-Tag system. These are the tags that are ascribed to the deficiencies in a facility. Some F-tags have been renumbered, others have moved or have been combined consistent with citations for new regulations.[52]

FIVE

A NEW PAYMENT MODEL

THE STORY OF J.A.

J.A. was initially a rather spry eight-five-year-old widowed gentleman who had been living in a skilled nursing facility for approximately five years; his long-term stay was covered by Medicaid. He had three married children, two of whom lived in other states while a third lived within an hour traveling distance. Because J.A. was beginning to become forgetful about simple daily routines, he was no longer able to live independently. His children, who were preoccupied with their own lives, made the decision for their dad to enter a nursing home. He was doing his best in the situation by making "friends" and participating in activities that interested him, albeit these were few.

As time went on, J.A. became less steady on his feet. At first he had to rely on using a cane. That progressed to a walker, and ultimately he was confined to a wheelchair. But J.A., who was now increasingly though pleasantly mildly confused, remembered when he was younger and more spry, able to walk independently to and fro within the facility, visiting his friends or going to the few activities he enjoyed. During these periods of confusion, he felt as though he were still that spry man and would attempt to get up from his wheelchair.

Of course, the result was several falls. Thankfully, up to now there had been no serious injuries. He would gently bump his head or shoulder as he fell. Each time he fell, it was reported to the physical therapist, who would assess the situation and usually schedule J.A. for therapy in an attempt to increase his strength and help him become more steady on his feet. If no one scheduled him for therapy, the physical therapist would collaborate with the nursing staff on interventions that would keep J.A. from falling. Some of them included making sure he was always near a staff member who could monitor him and remind him to sit back down when he attempted to stand (although due to the characteristic staff shortages within the facility, this was a difficult if not untenable plan) and ensuring he attended as many activities as possible to keep him engaged and occupied (although the activities were few and far between). Despite his being educated in the dangers of doing so, he repeatedly tried to get up and walk. Nurses, nurse aides, and other staff members and caregivers would gently remind him each time to sit down. After a while, that was the extent of their engagement with J. A. This is all too familiar for many individuals in nursing homes—and a disturbing scene for those of us who visit friends or family that "live" in them. (I put live in quotations, as describing this as living is a euphemistic term in these circumstances.) The sad part is, that after working in them for a while, most people become numb to the scene and consider it typical of the nursing home landscape. Mr. A. was relegated to sitting in the hall outside his room for most of the day, staring blankly at the drab, long hallway. His only contact with the staff was reduced to those times when he was being told to "sit down."

One particular nurse aides devised her own plan to provide one-on-one supervision for J.A. She would wheel him in his wheelchair with her from room to room, talking to him and engaging him in conversation while she went about her custodial duties of making beds and tidying up rooms. Of course, this was not a formalized "intervention," but one borne out of caring and compassion—a wonderful example of working with care in one's heart. The plan worked beautifully for the days and shifts this nurse aide worked with J.A. Seeing how well the plan worked, no one else, including the nurse manager of the floor, took the initiative to devise any other plans.

One day in mid-March, I was present when the occupational therapist reported to the physical therapist that J.A. had fallen once again. The physical therapist's response to the situation was both astonishing and appalling. He said, "I'll wait until he falls again and pick him up for therapy for CMI." (At that time CMI, or Case Mix Index, was a three-month period of time that occurred twice yearly when long-term residents with Medicaid coverage were scheduled for therapy to help ensure and increase the reimbursement rate for the facility.) Though Centers for Medicare & Medicaid Services has eliminated the Case Mix Index for calculating reimbursement, the example is provided to highlight how quality of care is compromised in favor of financial considerations.

The serious consequences are obvious. J.A.'s next fall, which in all probability was inevitable, could be much more serious. His fall could result in him having a stroke, breaking a hip, or incur injuries so severe they would result in his demise.

Whether it is a fall or some other accident, the facility is obliged to report the incident to an emergency contact or next of kin. In the unfortunate circumstance that you receive such a phone call, it would be prudent to ask the following questions:

1. What interventions have been implemented to ensure he/she is safer?

2. Was he/she evaluated and scheduled for therapy?

3. If he/she wasn't scheduled for therapy, why not?

It would also be prudent to request a copy of your loved one's medical record so you can see how the facility documented the incident and applied the remedies.

The Story of L.M.

LM. was a small, frail, and rather gaunt sixty-year-old resident who appeared much younger than his stated age. His large brown eyes bulged against his skin-and-bones appearance and extremely thin face. When anyone first came upon him in his room, they would not have expected that he had an ability to respond or communicate in any meaningful way. He had been diagnosed with a congenital neurologic deficit and was now dependent on a ventilator to breathe. However, when spoken to, he could blink his eyes to respond for yes or no and occasionally move his lips to form simple, short words in response to a basic question.

L.M. received all of his nutrition via a feeding tube. However, I was asked to see if it was possible for him to safely swallow anything by mouth. When I came to evaluate him, the occupational therapist was in his room working with him. She told me the physical therapist who had evaluated him had as a goal that he would be able to walk. Up until that point we had never even seen L.M. out of bed. We were definitely perplexed as his limbs and feet looked fairly contracted. Nevertheless, she proceeded to work with him and was able to get him to sit on the edge of the bed, a precursor to sitting in a chair or walking. After my course of therapy with L.M., it became clear he was unable to safely swallow food by mouth, but I continued to visit him from time to time to see if he was making any progress in other areas.

A few weeks went by, and then one day I heard from the director of another department that there were reports of L.M. walking. Neither of us could believe it, so we went to the unit to find out for ourselves. Indeed, the nurse on the unit reported that L.M. could now walk fifty feet. Astonished, and somewhat dismayed that no one had told me of this patient's progress which could have potential benefits to other areas of functioning, I went to the director of the rehabilitation department and asked about L.M.'s walking schedule so I could observe him. I explained that in my experience sometimes once people were upright and walking they also demonstrated an increased ability to safely swallow. I thought L.M. might be eligible for a reevaluation of his swallowing ability.

We arranged a day and time for me to observe. Because of his frail body and his attachment to the ventilator, three people were needed to assist him in that process—one on either side of him, one to guide the walker he would use, and one to follow with the wheelchair and appropriate ventilation equipment.

When the supervising physical therapist arrived to assist L.M., I was shocked by what he said. He announced that he wasn't sure how L.M. would do because it had been awhile since he last walked. But sure enough, with some effort and maximal assistance, L.M. walked from his room to the end of the hallway. Everyone cheered! What a feat!

Why did the physical therapist state it had been a while since L.M. had walked? Because he was scheduled for therapy for a specific period of time and purpose to maximize the financial gain to the facility. As mentioned earlier, that was known as the case mix index, or CMI, when the amount of therapy minutes for any one person was a crucial calculation for reimbursement. That's why after L.M. achieved the goal and was able to walk, therapy was discontinued and the facility did not provide any additional supportive programming. This is not only a horrendous abuse of the system, but also a severe blow to the resident who was able to achieve a level of function only to have it taken away. The facility was unwilling to expend money to have support staff continue to work with the resident, thus providing a higher quality of life. However, they "used" his therapy to receive a higher daily reimbursement rate. This is tragic for both the system and the resident.

———&&&———

The more information you have at your disposal regarding the inner workings of how a particular facility functions, and the more you can demonstrate your knowledge of that information by asking direct questions, the more cautious the facility will be about providing you with excuses and may be more inclined to ensure that the proper care is provided to your loved one. The expression, "the squeaky wheel gets the oil" definitely applies here. One of the situations facilities fear most is a family member who says they are aware of the improprieties and will report it to the Department of Health.

The Centers for Medicare and Medicaid Services, recognizing the pitfalls of the present system, took a bold step mid-year 2018 and eliminated the designated quarterly time period when residents would be evaluated and scheduled for therapy or other services in order to maximize reimbursement. The purpose of the overhaul was to address the widely known abuses and misuses of the system, close the loopholes used by ownership to maximize their reimbursement (essentially stop using the resident as a "piggy bank"), and reduce the overpayments which have been burdening the system. The new model, called the Patient Driven Payment Model, in concept is intended to be more driven by the patient's individual needs. This model disbands the use of the specific categories for therapy and skilled services which were prescribed in a way that converted to high scores used for calculating reimbursement. The new model also uses specific quarterly time periods; however, the facility will not know the dates of the quarter that will be captured. In this way, it is hoped that this will "encourage" facilities into providing treatment to residents as they are needed, as opposed to timing them to coincide with a specific time period. The method for calculating the reimbursement will be based on a checklist of categories in the booklet submitted to each respective state for reimbursement. Of course, the question arises: will some individuals be inclined to merely check off boxes on the forms submitted for reimbursement, whether or not the specific treatments or interventions have been applied? Will facilities choose to provide fewer rehabilitation services because they do not know what time frame is being viewed to calculate the reimbursement and therefore do not want to spend money on services for which they will not be reimbursed?

Yet the motivation behind creating such a system is obvious. Those that manipulated and bilked the system for financial gain, amassing large amounts of personal wealth without regard to true resident need, are the culprits. Since counting therapy minutes no longer affects reimbursement under this new system, the Centers for Medicare and Medicaid Services is aware of the potential adverse effect this may have on residents receiving the services they need and deserve. Therefore, they have stated that:

> If we discover that the amount of therapy provided to Skilled Nursing Facility residents does change significantly under the proposed Patient Driven Payment Model, if implemented, then we will assess the need for additional policies to ensure that Skilled Nursing Facility residents continue to receive sufficient and appropriate therapy services consistent with their unique needs and goals.[53]

Furthermore, since this new proposed model does not use therapy minutes to calculate reimbursement, there is concern that providers may attempt to mitigate their reduced reimbursement by providing therapy services in group or concurrent treatments, a practice that was abolished in 2011 as it was not considered to be an optimal model of service delivery. The Centers for Medicare and Medicaid Services is expected to closely monitor this situation and will consider denying coverage for facilities that violate this ruling. How could this be determined? If the number of patients treated and the number of therapy minutes provided by a therapist, exceeds the number of hours they have worked, this would clearly constitute a violation in this area.

PART THREE

WHERE ARE WE NOW?
WHAT IS POSSIBLE?
WHAT IS NEEDED?

SIX

THE FACE OF COMPASSIONATE CARE

Everybody Is Somebody

I have retold the following story many times throughout the years, mostly when I saw individuals being treated with a lack of compassion, respect, or empathy. I use it as an example that a small act and a few words can make a world of difference for someone.

I was working in a two hundred-bed facility in a very densely populated urban area. The brick building was sandwiched between many other buildings on a small, crowded inner-city side street. The streets were dirty, dusty, and noisy.

The first thing one noticed when entering the building was the shabby, somewhat dilapidated reception area. There were little or no attempts to dress it up to make it appear otherwise. The furniture in the small lobby was dated and stained. The reception desk was old, and the receptionist not entirely welcoming.

The residents of the building came from the surrounding area. Some had been "victims" of life and had been homeless prior to admission. Most of the other residents had worked at various menial jobs throughout their lives. What was particularly bothersome was the disdainful way the staff treated many of the residents. I could see the adage "everything starts at the top" play out right before my eyes. The dingy surroundings from the moment one stepped through the front door demonstrated the owners' lack of respect for both the workers and the residents. The attitudes of the staff toward the residents was an example of a complete trickle-down effect stemming from the attitude reflected in the rundown lobby.

On this particular day, I was working on a unit during the noon meal. I heard a resident calling out over and over from a small corner room. I was told by the staff that he was a problem resident and was always calling out. Not one staff member, not knowing if it was a serious matter, moved a muscle to find out the reason. I went to see if I could be of some help.

The resident was seated in a chair in his small room. His clothes were somewhat shabby and oversized for his small frame. I asked him what was wrong and he told me he just wanted another cup of coffee. I went and got the coffee and returned to the room, cup in hand. He said, "Thank you," and I responded, "My pleasure." I'll never forget the words he said in response; they brought tears to my eyes. He said, "Thank you—you make me feel like somebody." My heart sunk and I responded, "Everybody is somebody." He said sadly, "Not everybody acts that way."

What does it take for someone to feel as though they matter? In this situation, another person showing that they care about someone's needs and wants and just two small words: "My pleasure."

Everyone has a life story they want to share. It only takes a few minutes to listen.

My most recent foray was years later in a facility owned and operated by the same group as the one above. This facility was also in an urban area several blocks away from the other one, but it was a larger building with a more modern appearance from the outside. It was one block off a busy thoroughfare that was across the street from a large hospital complex. The block was not as crowded as the one where the previous facility was located, and therefore it had somewhat of a different feel.

Inside the front door was a small but neat reception area, with brightly painted walls, a few modern upholstered chairs, and a medium-sized enclosed bird aviary. The reception area was filled with the occasional chirping of the several small colorful birds flying back and forth. This is one of the reasons this building had different feel from the one I had worked in several years prior.

The units were typical of a nursing home. Long, lifeless, institutional-type hallways with fluorescent lighting and two-toned vinyl tiled floors. There were occasional private rooms, but most had two beds. In this facility, many members of the nursing staff were from a foreign country with a culture quite dissimilar from the culture of the residents in the local area. Though they spoke English, most had a pronounced foreign accent. Some had been in this country for several years; however, there were many who had come to the United States more recently. The nurse aides on the unit were from an entirely different culture than the nurses. Many of the staff members, especially the nurse aides, had worked in the facility for many years.

On this particular day, I received a doctor's order to evaluate a resident who returned from the hospital with a food consistency different from the one he was receiving prior to his hospitalization, which was regular.

I arrived on the unit to conduct a chart review and find out any pertinent information that might be helpful in my assessment of the resident's swallowing and food consistency. I was told: "He is cantankerous, belligerent, and rude" and I was warned to "be careful."

At that moment, I heard the wound doctor enter the room

to examine the resident. He did not knock first, and his approach seemed a bit abrupt. The resident quickly became loud and told the doctor he did not want to be examined.

Thinking it might not be a good idea to follow such an encounter, I left the unit and returned the following day. With his lunch tray in hand, I knocked on the door, as is required and obviously the considerate respectful thing to do when entering someone's private domain, and approached the man's bed. I introduced myself and told him I was here to evaluate his ability to eat regular food. Initially, he became loud and dismissive and said he did not want anything, waving his hand for me to remove his tray. I gently tried to explain my purpose again and told him how important it was for him to eat something. He said, "What's the use? They never send me what I want, and they always make mistakes." He picked up the meal ticket to show me that first of all, it did not include the foods he had requested, and secondly, some of the items on the tray were not what was written on the ticket. He said he was sick of it so he really couldn't be bothered with it anymore. He went on to say that the people in the kitchen didn't know how to do their jobs.

What I said to him next changed the entire dynamic of the conversation and his attitude from that moment forward. I told him that I'm sure if he did whatever job he had in the past, and made that many mistakes, he probably wouldn't have kept his job. I also told him there were no excuses for any of it. I assured him I would do whatever I could to correct the situation. This opened up a real conversation between us.

He told me he had been a doorman at a prestigious building in New York City for twenty-five years, and he mentioned some of the renowned people that lived there: a well-known past mayor of the city and a world-renowned anthropologist among them. He went on say how these people depended on him to take care of their deliveries and arrangements as needed. He was also proud to report that the owner of the building gave him special assignments. I listened intently and asked questions where it seemed relevant. The entire exchange took about ten minutes. But in that ten minutes, he had a chance to talk about what was so important to him in his life, how he rubbed elbows with famous people and was responsible for taking care of some of their day-to-day errands and needs. He felt validated and, with that interaction, he became more than just another body in a bed. He was a person that someone cared enough about to listen to and was interested in what he had to say.

From that moment forward he was more cooperative. I visited him from time to time, and whenever he saw me pass his room, he called out to me to say hello. He would even keep me abreast of how the kitchen was doing—when they did things right and when they made mistakes, but he did the latter in a far more affable manner. The nursing staff reported that his overall attitude had changed and he rarely had verbal outbursts.

Certainly, there are individuals whose disease process, situation, or personality results in them being cantankerous or verbally aggressive in some way. But it can also be the result of the lack of control they have over their environment and their life, dissatisfaction with things like food, having caregivers from foreign lands who they don't understand or who don't understand them, feeling abandoned by family, lonely and bored, and with the overall feeling that they never expected to wind up in such a situation. Instead of blaming such residents and labeling their behavior, caretakers and staff have to be aware of factors that may be affecting how they act. In this case, it took just a few minutes to show an interest in the resident's life . . . that he somehow had a purpose and a relevance before he came to the facility. That people regarded him, needed him—and that he mattered.

Acknowledging Someone *Does* Matter

I was covering for a colleague at a beautiful, local privately owned facility on sprawling grounds in an affluent suburb of a major city. It has been owned and operated by the same family for over fifty years. Immediately upon turning off the street to enter the property, one is struck by the beautifully landscaped grounds and overall vastness of the property. There were beds of beautifully colored flowers at the base of the pillars on each side of the drive. Atop the stone pillars were huge stone pots overflowing with various colored plants and flowers. All of this was surrounded by carefully planned shrubs and trees. I had been there several times over the years, and it has remained as beautiful as the first time I saw it. At the end of the long drive past the pillars, there is a large circular driveway that marks the facility entrance. In the middle of the circular driveway is a large, luxurious fountain surrounded by artfully arranged plants, shrubs, and flowers. The aroma from the flowers flowing gently in the breeze wafts through the air as you walk by to enter the doors of the facility. It is a sight befitting a mansion.

The 120 beds of the facility occupy only two floors; most of the patients come to the facility for short-term rehabilitation and are paying for their care privately. Many of them have also have private duty aides or companions that remain with them throughout the day and night. The majority of the patients also have frequent, if not daily, visits from family members.

The interior is as beautiful as the exterior. Each floor has two wings with mostly private rooms down three or four short hallways that extend from a central rotunda of sorts, albeit without the dome. This central area houses a spacious nursing station with patient charts. Here you will see nurses and other professionals doing their work with eyes glued to computer screens and papers strewn about. The scene is typical of what we identify with most nursing homes, though, maybe because of the vast space, it appears less frenetic. There are lots of windows throughout the building. On the sunniest of days, the sunlight brightens many of the hallways and one can almost feel the sun's warmth at almost every turn. At the end of most of the hallways are doors that lead to a small patio where patients are able to sit outside in the serene surroundings amongst the plants and flowers. One cannot help but admire the beautiful artwork on the hallway walls as well as the beautifully colored oil paintings in each room. Even more impressive are the several large bird cages on the upper floor that houses most of the short-term rehabilitation rooms. Large brightly colored parrots, cockatoos, and cockateels grace the cages. As you walk through the halls, you can hear birds chirping and parrots talking as they sometimes do. Occasionally staff members take the larger birds out of the cages and walk with them throughout the building; once in a while you'll see a patient with a bird perched on his or her shoulder. The lower floor mostly houses the long-term care residents, as well as the kitchen, laundry, and other essential services. While there are no birds on the lower floor, there is an outdoor central atrium with plants, shrubs, and a large cascading stone waterfall that lends a feeling of serenity to the area.

The staff is clearly trained to be polite and pleasant. Even staff members that I ran into from other facilities acted totally different in this environment. Everyone greets each other in the hallways, asks if they need help, and seems attentive to everyone's needs. This includes everyone from the top down—the director of nursing all the way to porters, laundry, and kitchen personnel and everyone in between. Interestingly enough, during my coverage this time around, I noticed that there were many more nurses from a foreign country.

However, despite the surroundings, the facility was still based on a medical model and one could not escape the "institutional" influence. Phones ringing, nurses bustling from place to place, and LPNs standing outside patient's room with their eyes either glued to the drawers of their medication carts as their fingers fiercely flicked one card after another to locate medications, or to the computer mounted atop the cart. And yet there was a feeling of calm throughout the building, even more so on the short-term rehabilitation floor. I attribute that to the spacious architectural design: the large windows and wide, sunlit hallways, the colorful birds, and the access to the outdoors.

On the second day I was at this facility, I went to see J.B., a patient assigned to the speech therapy program. He was seated in a wheelchair when I arrived. I introduced myself and pulled up a chair to sit next to him. J.B. was a rather tall man, and even with me seated next to him, he appeared to tower above me. He had a private duty aide who had been with him in his home for the past five years and remained with him during the day here. He had another private duty aide at night.

I had to explain the purpose of my visit to J.B. several times as he was somewhat confused and distractible. He seemed to finally understand. At that moment, the nurse came in to give him his medication. Being that he was apparently a confused gentleman, initially he was unwilling to open his mouth. She was also very tall and therefore seemed to be looming over him. I thought it would have been better if she attempted to address him at eye level rather than standing over him with a spoon in hand that was overloaded with applesauce containing crushed medication. In a rather hurried manner, she told she was there to give him his medication; she did not truly engage with him to make sure he understood what was expected. I also had to educate her about the appropriate amount to load on to the utensil in order to ensure the patient would swallow safely.

J.B. now had three people surrounding him: the private duty aide, me seated in a chair to his right, and the tall nurse looming over him with the spoon. It appeared that he could not make sense of the situation. Finally, through gentle coaxing, hand holding, and more explanation, he took the medication. Despite the beautiful surroundings and polite attitude of the staff in the hallways, the culture of patient care seemed to be typical of most other facilities.

The following day when I went to see J.B., he had been moved to a room on the lower level. Though there were approximately thirty beds for patients who would remain in the facility long-term on this unit, the plan for J.B. was definitely to return home. I had learned that the house where the patient lived with his wife was already outfitted with a hospital bed, the needed special equipment, and twenty-four-hour private duty assistance.

The next morning when I arrived at J.B.'s room for my scheduled session, the aide was on the phone with the patient's wife. The aide told her that her husband had not been changed for ten hours on the previous day and that when she went to tell the nurse at the nursing station, they replied that they were too busy. She told the wife that when she told them she would change him herself, she was told she was not authorized to do so. Once she got off the phone, she began to cry. She had been with J.B. for five years and cared for him deeply, and now she felt he wasn't getting the proper care. She also sensed that he was becoming increasingly physically uncomfortable. I comforted the aide, and J.B., upon seeing her cry, showed his concern. It was clear they had developed a bond. Despite the beautiful surroundings, some of what happened here was not so dissimilar to what happens in other traditional nursing homes.

Before I proceeded with my session, I told her during her next phone call with the patient's wife, she should advise her to call the director of nursing or the administrator.

Not more than five minutes later, the door opened abruptly without a knock. The director of nursing entered the room. Apparently J.B.'s wife had called her immediately after her conversation with the private duty aide. The nursing director walked directly up to the private aide without any greetings to anyone else in the room. She began questioning her extensively about the time frame that J.B. was not changed. The private duty aide was from a different culture, and had some difficulty understanding the director of nursing's questions. The convoluted questions were almost confusing to me. At one point, she told the aide that as the patient's advocate, it was her responsibility to insist that the patient receive the appropriate care. The aide was clearly reluctant to tell her that she had asked the nursing staff to have someone attend to the patient but their response was that they were short-staffed and too busy. At the conclusion of her dialogue with the aide, the director promised that she would speak with the staff. Then she left the room.

Mr. J.B. was seated upright in bed. Because of his height, I was standing next to him so I could be at his eye level while assisting him with eating. As soon as the director of nursing left the room, he looked at me blankly and said, "Who was that? What was she doing here, and what was she talking about?" Despite the fact that J.B. was easily confused, the director of nursing never greeted him, addressed him, or even looked at him. She was talking about him, but it was as though he wasn't even there. Clearly, he was aware enough to know that he hadn't been treated as if he were there or as if he mattered at all. If the director of nursing acted this way toward a patient, how would the rest of her nursing staff be expected to behave toward patients? The incongruity of the situation was stunning. In this facility, the staff was trained to great each other in the hallways and express "apparent" interest and concern for anyone they came upon. However, once again, as had been the case for Mr. J.B. the previous day, it wasn't always reflected in the care patients received.

I also noted another disturbing situation in this facility while observing patients during mealtimes. The nursing aides were not providing the necessary assistance for some of the older patients who received regular consistency food. Much of the larger pieces of food were presented to the residents without being cut. I mentioned this to the director of the rehabilitation department, who also served as the facility's assistant administrator. I explained that I observed patients coughing as a result of placing overly large pieces of uncut food in their mouths, creating a potential for choking. She responded in a rather dismissive fashion and actually seemed unconcerned about the seriousness of the matter. She did tell me there had been numerous staff training sessions, but to no avail.

It seemed counterintuitive that a facility in which the staff was successfully trained to greet each person they come upon in the hallway with the utmost politeness and respect was unable to successfully train the staff to cut people's food into bite-sized pieces. How many of the patients actually required this level of assistance, especially since many of them had private duty aides in attendance with them throughout the day? This is a relatively small facility of just 120 people, the majority of whom were alert and physically capable, merely needing rehabilitation for a broken hip, knee replacement, shoulder or back issue, or a cardiac problem, etc. Where was the oversight to insist that they were fed properly? Who conducted dining room rounds?

I continued talking with the director of rehabilitation about compassion and empathy in patient care. She responded that they had looked at all of the issues but hadn't been successful. She used the example of staff knocking on a patient's door, then rushing in and out to complete their assigned tasks with little quality interaction with the patient. She told me that staff turnover was part of the problem. I said that if the expectation was for staff members to be polite and respectful in the hallway, then they could also be trained to treat patients with more empathy. She told me the staff could not be trained in the areas of improved communication and empathy with patients/residents. Of course, I disagreed. However, being that I was only covering in this facility for a few days, I could not pursue the matter as I normally would with a director of nursing and/or administrator. .

Later that day I was treating one of my patients whose daughter was in attendance. The daughter told me about some of her dissatisfactions with this beautiful facility—for example, something as simple as having her mother's dentures applied with adhesive so that they remain securely in place. She used two words to convey her impression of the facility: window dressing. Considering some of what I experienced, I thought they were very appropriate.

The above examples are a few, among many, that happen every day in almost every nursing home across the country.

What do these stories have in common?

The fact that despite the surroundings—whether inner city or sprawling suburb—there is a need for greater understanding of how to treat, care for, and talk with patients.

An Example of Empathetic Care:
It Starts at the Top and Makes a Big Difference

My experience from the many facilities in which I have worked is that workers feel that the administration or ownership doesn't care about them. They feel they are little more than a warm body filling a role to do a job that needs to be done. The "trickle down" effect is that many workers do their jobs in ways that are equally "uncaring."

What would it take for the administration to show workers they are valued? To the casual onlooker, this following example may seem like a small and insignificant gesture. To many it might have even gone unnoticed. But it made a big difference in the lives and attitudes of the workers in this facility, and in turn, an even bigger difference for the residents.

In a facility I worked in many years ago, each day the owner made "rounds" with the administrator, meaning that the two of them walked through each unit in the building. One day shortly after I began working at the facility, I came upon the owner in the hallway. He approached me, introduced himself, and asked my name and my role in the building. We chatted for a few minutes before he continued walking down the hallway. I had never experienced that before. My experience up to that point was that owners (as well as administrators) would walk past me without even a hello or a glance in my direction. They would walk through the halls, barely looking at anyone, sometimes even looking past people as if they didn't exist. They only address the people they see as being important: a doctor, a nurse manager, another department head. That's why this owner made such a strong impression on me. As I watched him continue his rounds, he frequently stopped to speak with both the residents and workers. He knew each worker's name, as well as pertinent information about them. He would ask about their vacations, their children's birthday or graduation, or a family member's illness. It was no wonder that the workers in this facility seemed to love coming to work and had a sense of commitment to their residents, their coworkers, and the facility in general. This facility had a very low rate of staff turnover.

What Does It Really Take to Change the Culture?

It's probably unrealistic to think that owners will independently come to the realization that empathic care is an important ingredient for an improved quality of life and the overall satisfaction residents experience within a facility. It will also probably not occur solely as a result of changes enacted by regulatory bodies. Here are two ingredients for cultural change:

1. Changing Attitudes. First and foremost, it requires changing attitudes from the way people are often treated to ones that convey respect and empathy. This, first and foremost, can begin to affect a shift in how a person feels about themselves and about being in a facility. However, this also stems from the respect and value the administration places on those individuals who work in the facility and are charged with caring for the people who reside in them. Management that views and treats workers as more than "warm bodies" would probably have more success in their attitude towards the people for whom they care. This would involve taking an interest in the quality of the individual and their experience, philosophy, and attitude about working with people who reside in nursing homes. Everything is systemic and starts at the top; this would go a long way to creating attitude change.

2. Fair Wages for Hourly Workers. I contend that a fair hourly wage for the workers, especially Certified Nursing Assistants who are responsible for caring for individuals on a daily basis, is an important step. Many workers struggle financially to the point that they are relegated to living with relatives or living in a homeless shelter. This is unacceptable. Being valued and treated with respect and dignity from an employer can go a long way in showing respect and dignity for others, and appropriate compensation is an important ingredient.

Empathy as the New Face of Compassionate Care

Compassion is a feeling of sympathy for the suffering and misfortune of others that comes from a person's own heart. Some people have more compassion than others. *Empathy* is actually feeling what it means to be in someone's situation and conveying that to them. It's an understanding of what it would be like to be in their shoes, to feel what they may be going through, and share or validate a variety of the emotions they may be feeling (i.e., fear, anxiety, pain, worry, loneliness, abandonment, boredom, loss of independence). It has been proven that when care is rendered in a more empathetic fashion, both the patient and the caregiver experience greater satisfaction.

Empathy in Practice

If you want to see an exemplary example of empathy in practice, in this episode of *The View,* Vice President Joe Biden comforts Meghan McCain as she talks about her father's brain cancer. How did he convey empathy? By getting up, sitting next to her, looking in her eye, giving her a comforting touch, and speaking to her in a very personal way. There is a strong communication component when expressing empathy.[54]

Empathy is being increasingly recognized as an important component in patient care. Toward this end, medical, nursing schools and hospitals are adding empathy training to their curriculum and orientation programs. Studies have shown that physicians who participated in empathy training had an improved ability to make their patients feel more at ease and developed a better understanding of them and their problems. This led to an improved physician-patient connection that then resulted in improved patient satisfaction. As a result, patients were more likely to comply with their treatments, resulting in better outcomes.

The counter-argument from those who object is that "empathizing" with each patient will take too much time. Schedules rooted in a business medical model are geared for maximizing revenue and are already crunched for time. However, that objection has been negated by Dr. Helen Reiss, a physician at Massachusetts General Hospital,[55] who reported that physicians can more easily and quickly determine a patient's issues if they express more empathy. The article also reports that many malpractice cases are the result of miscommunication. Therefore, improved empathy can potentially reduce the risk of malpractice. An added benefit for the physician is a reduction in physician burnout.

With medical schools, nursing schools, and hospitals embracing the importance of empathy training, it seems that skilled nursing facilities should be coming to the same conclusion. It's even more critical in the case of patients with Alzheimer's disease or dementia.

The Robot Solution or Artificial Intelligence: A Viable Alternative?

As mentioned in chapter 2, at 26.3 percent, Japan has the highest percentage of people over the age of sixty-five in the world. With the growing population of older people, loneliness has become a widespread concern and has grown to epidemic proportions as young people move to more urban areas for work and work extremely long hours. This results in people having little time for social lives, their own partners and children, and their elders.

Statistics estimate that there are 18.4 million adults living alone in Japan, with projections that by the year 2040, the percentage of those living alone will jump to 40 percent. The result has been something known as *kodokushi*: people dying alone and remaining undiscovered for long periods of time. Some estimate that thirty thousand people die alone each year; however, there are other reports that the number can be twice or three times higher than that.[56]

This "epidemic" has created a public health concern that has been linked to depression, dementia, and heart disease. To fill the human need for communication and social contact, the technology industry stepped up and developed a robotic seal called Paro as a substitute. These robotic seals are being provided, not only to people in their homes, but also in care facilities as a means of providing therapy and social interactions. Residents can talk or sing to the "seals" and have been seen picking them up and hugging them. The seal responds by looking up, blinking, and making gentle cooing noises.

A facility known as Silver Wing Care Facility utilizes a more humanoid robot called Pepper to direct a midday exercise session. This more "humanoid"-designed robot has even been "adopted" by families as a substitute for children or grandchildren.[57]

Japan continues to be on the cutting edge of robotic advancements for nursing care as a response to the need created by the surge in the older population. They developed a robot called ROBEAR to lift patients from a bed into a wheelchair or to help them stand. ROBEAR was called the "strong robot with the gentle touch."[58]

"There is now strong evidence relating greater depressive symptoms to increased progression from normal cognition to mild cognitive impairment and from mild cognitive impairment to dementia," according to Dr. Donovan and his colleagues. They suggest that loneliness, as well as low-grade and more serious depression, may have similar pathological effects on the brain—all of which raises the question of how loneliness and social isolation might be countered to help ward off cognitive decline and other adverse health effects.[59]

While this may be applicable to situations where people are living independently, loneliness and boredom are hallmarks of life in nursing home facilities. Thus, we need to take notice and design facilities with programs to address these issues rather than resorting to prescribing drugs as the solution.

Companies in the U.S. also are experimenting with robot caregivers. In 2011, HStar Technologies, a Massachusetts-based company, received a $1.5 million grant from the Small Business Research Innovation program to develop the robotic nursing assistant known as RoNA.[60] The project was conceived to prevent back injuries while carrying or helping to turn or lift patients in bed, especially those patients of a heavier weight. RoNA has been used in hospitals and care facilities as well as for assisting the military in combat zones.

What is your reaction to all this? Are we now going to use robots to care for patients? Are we going to remove the remaining human element from medical care? Robots and caretaking or caregiving seem to me to be contradictory ideas. That was my reaction at first. But after thinking about it for a greater length of time, I realized that using robotics presents an interesting notion.

Using robots to assist caregivers can surely save them from potential injuries, especially back injuries which they may experience when turning and lifting patients of a heavier weight. But is can also improve efficiency by ensuring that tasks are completed and recorded accurately. When considered together, these may seem like a logical reason for their use. Nursing aides still have to record tasks after completion, leaving the possibility for error. And too often tasks are recorded without first being completed to the obvious detriment of the patient. (Turning patients according to a prescribed schedule is only one small example.)

The cost saving component of a robotic nursing assistant cannot be ignored. It could allow for nursing aides to care for more patients in less time, which could also allow them more time for human interaction and compassionate care. Of course, in order for this to take place, owners would have to recognize and value the importance of empathy in care, which would involve a shift away from the present thinking. The desire to increase profits might lead some facilities to merely add more patients to the workload because of the efficiency afforded them with the use of a robotic nursing assistant.

Will the United Sates take Japan's example and seriously consider incorporating robots into facilities to fulfill or augment the role of a nursing assistant? A personal friend of mine is an executive with a small company that owns and operates nursing homes. We recently discussed the use of robots in nursing homes, and he told me there is concern about the public reaction to rolling them out for use.

There are, of course, additional considerations. Union issues would have to be addressed with possible changes in job descriptions. Additional training would be required to teach people how to interact with robots. The Centers for Medicare and Medicaid Services would have to reexamine staffing requirements, an issue they have yet to address, and consider the role of robotic nursing assistants in their nursing home regulations. How would annual surveys address or judge the use and care of robots in a facility?

Here are some of the questions and concerns that I have. You may have others.

- Are there any studies on how patients, especially older and/or confused patients, would respond to a robot?
- Are there any plans to use a robotic nursing assistant in a long-term care facility as a test case?
- Is a more humanoid-looking robot in development? ROBEAR is almost a caricature, but we certainly have seen enough movies with human-looking robots.
- How will patients respond to a humanoid-looking machine? Considering the ever-growing population with Alzheimer's, will robots be used with these individuals as well?
- Can the robot be programmed to be empathetic? What about if the patient is not ready or willing to get up at that time? Will the robot be able to determine that and be able to adjust its response?
- Will the robot be able to sense a decline in a patient?
- Will owners try to circumvent the issues surrounding the cost of human nursing assistants and hire more robots to do tasks? Will there be sufficient oversight to ensure this does not happen?
- Will robots be "assigned" to work with patients with specific or a wide range of deficits? Will there be limits applied to the use of robots?
- Will the robot speak? How will the robot be programmed to speak with patients in a multicultural society in which people speak different languages?

- How would a robot respond if a patient acts out by being physically or verbally aggressive?

- How far along is the research?

- Who will oversee the robots' effectiveness?

- Who will oversee the mechanical functioning of the robots? (This might require developing an entire new tech industry for facilities and hospitals.) How scientifically advanced would someone have to be to service the robot in the event of a malfunction?

- Do robots need periodic servicing? Sometimes it's hard enough to have a tech person remedy a desktop or laptop issue.

- What about the need for human touch? How will patients respond to a robotic touch? Does it fill the same need?

A recent experience prompted me to think about this even further. I attempted to reach the technical repair center of a major television provider when a channel on my TV stopped working in the midst of viewing a major sporting event. I made several attempts to reach a live person, but each time I contacted the provider, I received a computer-generated voice that insisted I could speak to it in complete sentences and it could help solve my problem. Of course, the preprogrammed options and solutions were not applicable to the problem I was experiencing; I'm sure many people reading this have had similar experiences.

I tried everything I could think of, including repeatedly pressing "0," thinking this might trigger the system to transfer me to a live person. Since repeating the word *representative* over and over had worked in other situations for other companies, I tried that as well, to no avail. I hung up and called again at least four times, hoping to finally reach a live person, but that did not get me any success either. This went on for approximately thirty minutes. It was maddening, my frustration mounted, and I felt like screaming! And this was only related to reception of a channel on a TV set.

This led me to think about how a robot would respond to questions or situations outside the realm for which it was programmed. It would be interacting with human beings, some capable of expressing themselves but many others unable to do so. How would this affect the individual who has already experienced a loss of independence, autonomy, and friends and family by being confined to a nursing home facility?

Compassion comes from the heart, and although one might think that is what drives people to work in this industry, this is not entirely the case. Some people merely see it as a job. I have been saying for many years that people are working, but they work without heart. I recently read a statement by a resident of a facility who stated it somewhat differently but I think perfectly: "When there is care in the heart, you can see it in the help." I may also add that you can *feel* it in the help.

Because I have heard claims that there is a shortage of health care workers that will continue as the aging population grows, individuals are hired irrespective of any litmus test about their capacity to render care with compassion or empathy. In addition, the strain of being short-staffed and the pressure to complete assignments in a prescribed period of time for an ever-growing number of patients each day causes staff to minimize their interactions with residents. Less time, less interaction, less opportunity to care with empathy or convey compassion—the result is that our loved ones feel less cared about and the professional is less interested and less invested in the treatment outcome.

We are social beings. The need for physical contact and verbal communication with others is well documented. The absence of it leads to loneliness, depression, and withdrawal that are also hallmarks of nursing home existence. It is a contradiction in terms that people move from living independently because they are no longer able to do so, or because they are isolated and alone, to an environment where they are surrounded by people and yet become lonely, depressed, and withdrawn.

SEVEN

TRAILBLAZING ALTERNATIVES TO LONG-TERM CARE NURSING HOMES

WHO DO WE SEE?

There he was, seated in a wheelchair, the right side of his face and mouth obviously drooping. He began to speak. The words were few and the sentences short. His speech was slow, somewhat slurred, and appeared to take great effort, but with careful listening, it could be understood. The voice sounded vaguely familiar, but his face was somewhat difficult to recognize.

He had a severe stroke a little over twenty years ago at the end of January 1996. At that time the doctors told his wife he most likely had lost the ability to speak. Not one to give up or be silenced, he endured daily speech therapy sessions for several months. Finally, he did regain the ability to express simple ideas using short, simple sentences. He had to speak slowly in order to be understood.

Now he is 101 years old. He had been an intense man with an extraordinarily successful career. One could hardly see that now. To the casual observer, not knowing his history, he was just an old man with impaired speech sitting in a wheelchair.

Sunday, January 7, 2018. The audience erupts in applause. They rise to their feet, cheering wildly. The uproarious ovation reaches a crescendo that goes on for several minutes until the audience is finally quieted and returns to their seats.

It is the nationally televised *Golden Globe Awards*. Who was this "old man" in the wheelchair that inspired such resounding acclaim? None other than one of the greatest actors of our time, Kirk Douglas.

The casual observer who might not know this motion picture legend would only see a 101-year-old man in a wheelchair with slurred and limited speech. Like so many other elder citizens in the community, in assisted living facilities, or in skilled nursing facilities, they would probably pass him by without a thought about his life, his achievements, his greatness, and they would pay little attention to anything he had to say.

I recently inadvertently received some photos of legendary actors—specifically, Doris Day and Gene Hackman. I couldn't believe how they looked now as compared to how they looked in their youth. The aging process treats us all the same. Yes, we say some people age better than others. But, after a certain age, the changes catch up to us in similar ways. I thought to myself, *I wonder if other people would have the same reaction.* I invite you to enter the names of well-known or favorite actors or political figures into your preferred search engine browser to view pictures of them, now and then. Be honest as you ask yourself this question. If you did not know who they were, would your perception of them change?

Would you just view them as another "elderly" or "old" person and look away, pass them by, or not want to be bothered or give them the time of day? Or would you give them more credence because you know who they are, or were?

Do these legendary actors deserve more notice because of their celebrity?

So, what of our elder citizens who are unknown to us through celebrity or the political arena? Those individuals who you might just pass on the street or are out of plain sight because of where they are living?

Doesn't each person have importance in the lives of their own family, in their own life, on whatever level? Is that not to be recognized? Should we pass them by, or look askance at them, or ignore them as if they are not there? As if they don't matter? As if they no longer exist?

There have been a variety of alternatives to the traditional nursing home/skilled nursing facility model developed in the 1980s. Yet, despite the initial success and growth of facilities that embody a more humanistic approach to caring for our elder citizens, the traditional models continue to thrive, and the corporatization of the nursing home industry with the traditional structure continues to grow. This is a *very sad fact.*

Is it only because it is easier, more expedient, and, above all, more profitable? While it may not be practical to imagine that the over 15,000 traditional nursing homes across the country could be revamped to represent an alternative model, it is my premise that even if small changes can be incorporated into the present system, there is a real chance that those who find themselves in such places will be treated with greater dignity, respect, and care, and, therefore, experience an improved quality of life. During my research, I came across an article by Alana Samuels published in *The Atlantic* in April 2015. It stated the exact same information I had written. "After plenty of isolated successes, the question isn't what good nursing homes look like, but how to transform existing facilities into places that look like them."[61] This is especially important considering the continued growth of our older population and the increased numbers of those afflicted with Alzheimer's disease.

It is useful to look at the existing successful models and what they have been able to achieve. I have been inspired by them, and I hope you will be as well. They share many innovative solutions in common, but each presented with its own unique style.

PARK PLACE—Portland, Oregon

One of the first innovators in the area of eldercare was Keren Brown Wilson. The story begins when she was a young child. Her father died suddenly, and her mother suffered a debilitating stroke at the age of fifty-five when Keren was in college. The stroke left her mother paralyzed on one side of her body, unable to walk. Her face was also paralyzed and drooped on one side, a common occurrence when one suffers a stroke, and her speech was slurred. This in no way affected her ability to think clearly or express herself adequately—a situation that many victims of strokes, and their families, find particularly frustrating. The body has failed, but the mind has not.

Because of her physical limitations, Keren's mother was unable to care for herself and there wasn't any money for outside help. Her mother was a poor woman who was now receiving Medicaid. Keren, a college student, didn't have an income and lived in a small apartment with a roommate. She had other siblings, but their circumstances were also not suitable for taking care of their mother.

There was unfortunately only one choice: a nursing home. Keren opted for one nearby her school. Though it seemed like a "nice enough" place, her mother always begged her to "get me out of here." Probably as a result of her mother's plight, Keren became interested in policy for the aged and pursued this in her studies. After graduating, she landed a job in Washington, working in the area of senior services. Her mother moved to a variety of nursing homes, nearby one or another of her children. Keren eventually married. Her husband, a sociologist, encouraged her to continue her studies toward earning a PhD, which she did. After graduating, she decided to work on the science of aging. When she told her mother of her plans, her mother asked her a question which was the inspiration that took her life in a completely different and unexpected direction: "Why aren't you doing something to help people like me?"

Atul Gawande, in his book *Being Mortal,* writes about Keren Brown Wilson's story and her mother's vision:

> She wanted a small place with a little kitchen and a bathroom. It would have her favorite things in it, including her cat, unfinished projects, her Vicks VapoRub, a coffeepot, and cigarettes. There would be people to help her with the things she couldn't do for herself. In the place she imagined, she would be able to lock her own door, control the temperature, and have her own furniture. There would be no one to make her get up when she didn't want to, turn off her favorite soap operas, or ruin her clothes. They wouldn't be able to throw away the back issues of magazines or "treasures" she collected from Goodwill because they created clutter and a safety hazard. She could have privacy whenever she wanted, and no one could make her get dressed if she didn't feel like it, take her medicine, or go to activities she didn't like. She would feel like a person rather than some anonymous patient in a bed.[62]

This description is certainly in sharp contrast to the nursing homes we know that are essentially watered-down versions of a hospital—the kind of nursing home I have been talking about throughout the book. These typically comprise long, lifeless, sterile, vinyl-floored hallways with some single but mostly double-bedded rooms (some also have three- and four-bedded rooms).

Along the hallways, residents sit in their wheelchairs, appearing almost lifeless, expressionless, bored, with a vacant look in their eyes. Other residents remain lying in their beds. Some are actually crying out for help. It is a rather disturbing sight, and one we have all come to think of as characteristic of a nursing home environment.

There is usually also a central nursing station with the constant beep of clanging bells and ringing phones, and in some cases repeated overhead pages.

It should be noted that overhead paging is now acknowledged as an intrusion into the daily lives of the residents living in a facility (which is essentially their home). In recent years many facilities are opting to use text messaging with facility-issued phones in order for staff members to communicate with one another. Use of overhead pages are reserved for emergencies.

Some facilities make an effort to pretend that they are something other than they are by calling each unit a "community" or "neighborhood" and giving them cute, fun names. This does nothing to change the stark reality of what they are in actuality. Keren Brown Wilson described the nursing homes that her mother was in.

> Nursing homes were really stripped-down hospitals. People were in a ward. They were literally in a bed. They were told when to go to bed. They were told when to get up. They were told what to eat. They were told what they could do and what they couldn't do—and they really had no autonomy. They had no say in their lives. And that was very dehumanizing.[63]

Despite the fact that the conventional thinking was that it would be unsafe for elder citizens to live more independently and have more autonomy over their own lives, Keren Brown Wilson, together with her husband, found a way to borrow millions of dollars to help build their mother's vision of what they themselves also believed was possible. She thought that just because a person was old and frail, it didn't mean they essentially should be locked away in an institution-like fortress where they were forced to give up their rights to an independent life. Their vision was to create a homelike atmosphere where individuals would be free to make their own decisions about how to spend their time, what they did in their own space, and the possessions they chose to have. They could determine their own "lights out" and rising times and what they wanted to eat. Wilson and her husband had to overcome countless obstacles and resistance from both the public policy makers and the political sector.

Eventually, after receiving financial backing from a private donor, they succeeded in bringing their vision to life, and in 1983 they developed Park Place in Portland, Oregon, a model of assisted living for the elderly. It was one of the first of its kind in the United States.

> No one really believed it could be done. And no one thought that we could give nursing care in a non-nursing setting. No one believed that people would be safe. I mean people were convinced that it would kill people.[64]

These facilities were able to serve those with lower incomes at a flat rate, and it showed that their health outcomes were better than those living in traditional nursing homes. This new model of care for the elderly attracted the attention of the national media, and it received widespread acclaim. Wilson and her husband were able to replicate the initial project with several other assisted living centers throughout Oregon. Eventually, they formed a company called Assisted Living Concept, and with the backing of Wall Street investors, Keren Brown Wilson was able to take her vision public. It gave way to the birth of other assisted living companies with names that may sound familiar: Sunrise, Atria, Sterling, and Karrington. During the next several years, she was able to oversee the building of hundreds of assisted living facilities across eighteen states throughout the country. By 2010, the number of people living in assisted living facilities was approaching the number living in nursing homes. This now serves as a model for eldercare worldwide.

Keren Brown Wilson now focuses on developing sustainable programs to meet the basic needs of elder citizens without sufficient income, especially in the area where she grew up, the coal mining hills of West Virginia. She is president of the Jessie F. Richardson Foundation, named after her mother, and heads the Aging Matters Initiative. In her role at these two organizations, her work addresses the important issues related to housing and services for the older population whose income or lack thereof places them at risk. Her work extends beyond the United States to Central America.

CHASE MEMORIAL NURSING HOME—New Berlin, New York

Bill Thomas is from a small town in upstate New York. He went off to Harvard as a young man to study medicine. He had every opportunity to become a prosperous and successful doctor in a thriving metropolis, but his heart was always with his hometown, New Berlin. He initially worked as a doctor in emergency medicine before becoming medical director for a small local nursing home, Chase Memorial. He was thirty-one years old, with little experience in nursing home care, except for his residency in family medicine. The nursing home had a combination of residents ranging from the severely disabled to those with cognitive impairment as a result of Alzheimer's disease. As with most people who enter a nursing home, Bill Thomas found it to be an extremely depressing environment with dreary surroundings, a lackluster environment giving way to lackluster lives. His initial instincts were to prescribe treatments to address what he thought might be the underlying cause. He prescribed numerous tests, x-rays, specialist appointments, and ultimately prescription medications, but none of these effected any significant change.

Having grown up in rural, upstate New York, it struck Dr. Thomas that life on a farm—in particular the need to take care of other living things, whether plants or animals—could possibly be the missing ingredient needed in the nursing home: life itself. He developed a proposal to bring life in every form into the nursing home: dogs, cats, birds, and plants. His proposal was massive—two dogs for each of the two floors, two cats for each floor, and plants and birds, one hundred of them. But these animals did not casually "pass through" on a particular schedule as happens in many facilities. They lived in the building. He also wanted to develop a program to have children become part of the daily lives and fabric of the nursing home. He personally lobbied lawmakers in Albany to obtain the necessary approvals and present his grant proposal. He was successful in both areas.

Implementing such a grandiose plan was not easy. As one could imagine, there was resistance on many levels. Yet this small facility is now full of dogs, cats, birds, and plants galore. Understandably, some of the resistance came from professional staff members who were faced with a newfound role—caring for and feeding pets—certainly not formerly part of their professional responsibility.

In my profession, I have found that introducing new speech or dysphagia therapy programs, or new diet consistencies have been problematic. The resistance and pushback can be unbelievably strong, and these are programs that *are* the very fabric of ensuring resident safety and well-being. At times I have felt like a fish swimming upstream against fierce currents, even with support from administration, rehabilitation department directors, and directors of nursing. I can only imagine how it must have been for Bill Thomas introducing this menagerie of animals and plants. But Dr. Thomas had an indomitable spirit, and he was undeterred.

Transformations began to happen. That is probably what finally turned the tide in peoples' attitudes. Residents who hadn't spoken began to speak. People who hadn't been walking suddenly began asking if they could take the dog for a walk. The parakeets were adopted and given names. The menagerie of animals grew to include rabbits and egg-laying hens.

This change in peoples' behavior was demonstrated as early as the 1970s in a study by Judith Rodin and Ellen Langer.[65] They divided residents into two groups. The first group was given autonomy over their lives and surroundings. They were allowed to arrange the furniture in their rooms any way they liked, go where they wanted, and do what they wanted with whom they wanted. Each person was also given a plant to water and care for. Isn't this what we do in our own everyday lives? The second group was told that the staff was there to care for them and water the plant. The result of the eighteen-month long study bears out what happened at Chase Memorial. The residents in group one who were able to exercise autonomy over their lives and had responsibility for the plant demonstrated improved health. There was little to no change for the residents in group two, and there was an increased proportion in the number of deaths.

A comparative study of the residents of Chase Memorial with another local nursing home over a two-year period revealed astonishing results. The number of prescription drugs needed fell by one-half, especially the need for psychotropic medications like Haldol. Total pharmacy bill costs fell to just 38 percent of the other facility, and deaths decreased by 1.5 percent.

THE GREEN HOUSE PROJECT—THE EDEN ALTERNATIVE

In 2000, Bill Thomas wanted to build a nursing home from the ground up that would incorporate what he learned from Chase Memorial Home. He wanted it to be affordable and able to accept Medicaid patients, but he did not want it to have the look of being built with that kind of budgetary consideration. Of course, it was essential that it have a homelike feel as opposed to a hospital. An organization in Tupelo, Mississippi, agreed to build what came to be known as "Green Houses." Each home had ten to twelve private bedrooms with private bathrooms and was arranged around communal living areas and kitchen.

The residents, known as elders, were also involved in planning their own menus. There is a strong difference in culture and attitude in these Green Houses. The person-centered care with its emphasis on team building and leadership provides greater satisfaction, greater sense of community, and more involvement from both staff and residents/elders. Each of the homes has a primary caregiver, who has essentially the same role as a certified nurse's aide; however, this person is called a Shahbaz.[66] These staff members also provide housekeeping tasks such as room cleaning and laundry and help residents plan activities. The Shahbaz has a supervisor known as a Guide who essentially oversees the home's operations. Each home also has a resident representative known as the Sage. This is similar to a representative of a resident council in a traditional nursing home facility. The Sage volunteers to be a mentor and advisor to the work teams in the home. There is a clinical support team consisting of nurses, therapists, ancillary services, activities, and dietitians who provide services as needed. This team works with the Shahbaz to provide individualized care for each elder, similar to individualized care plans developed in the traditional setting.

Studies found that residents who lived in these Green Houses were happier and experienced a better quality of life. Furthermore, staff members were more satisfied with their jobs, and there was less staff turnover. Staff reported feeling less rushed, less stressed, and less guilty.

The Robert Wood Johnson Foundation in 2005 funded a five-year grant program in the United States to develop what is now known as the Green House Project. It is a nonprofit organization, the purpose of which was to develop and build alternatives to the traditional nursing home facilities at various locations throughout the United States. After the initial five-year grant, the project continued.

As of February 2015, there were 174 Green Houses on forty campuses operating in twenty-seven states, and another 186 in development.[67] Government agencies have become aware of the benefits of Green Houses, and this led the public housing authority in Loveland, Colorado, to build a Green House. Residents who live in a Green House experience more privacy, autonomy, satisfaction with food and a higher level of dignity. There is evidence that residents who live in Green House Project homes demonstrate increased mobility, have more social interactions, and there are fewer reports of weight loss and depression.[68]

There are currently studies being conducted to determine the costs to Medicare and Medicaid for residents in Green Houses as compared with traditional nursing homes. Though there have not been any sweeping reports to date, certain states indicate that there is parity between the two. Green House Project homes may be licensed as traditional nursing homes and, as such, are eligible to receive Medicaid and Medicare reimbursements consistent with the traditional nursing home facilities.

A 2004 report presented to the United States Congress from researchers at the School of Public Health at the University of Minnesota found that a more socialized model of care along with empowering staff to serve those elders who needed skilled nursing care demonstrated statistically significant, favorable outcomes over traditional facilities.[69] In November 2008, Max Baucus (D-MT), chairman of the Senate Finance Committee, said that the Green House Project model "has shown promise for both improving the quality of life and care in these settings."[70]

The Green House concept is not solely about the architectural design. It is based on a philosophy about prioritizing the individual and providing compassionate and respectful care. This is the concept at the heart of the design. The Green House Project is now dedicated to finding a way to change how the more traditional institutional homes function. This new initiative is known as the "Pathway to Green House."

THE LEONARD FLORENCE CENTER FOR LIVING GREEN HOUSE—Chelsea, Massachusetts

The story behind the Leonard Florence Center for Living is one that I think should be highly publicized in the hopes of inspiring a change throughout the nursing home industry.

It is the story of Barry Berman's mother, who was placed in the nursing home that he himself directed after she suffered a massive stroke and had a bout with pneumonia. He was confident the facility would treat his mother well; they were known to be efficient and provide good care. However, after a few days he went to visit his mom and couldn't believe his eyes.

> I'll never forget the feeling as long as I live. I said, "Oh my God, there's my mother, this old woman, in a wheelchair, lifeless. Look what my own nursing home did to my own mother in a matter of days."[71]

Prior to this, Mr. Berman had been a director of both assisted living and nursing home complexes over a period of twenty-three years. However, in this instance, he was unable to help his own mother, and he came face-to-face with the harsh reality of what the nursing home environment meant to an elderly person. Needless to say, he immediately moved his mother out of the facility and arranged for health aides to care for her at home. Afterward he proceeded to completely transform the way the Chelsea Jewish Foundation, which he directed, cared for their elderly patients. He then embarked on a project to build a home that would look totally different than the institutional environment of the traditional nursing home.

He based this new facility on an innovative experiment known as the Eden Alternative, and in 2010 the Leonard Florence Center for Living Green House opened. It is an award-winning, state-of-the-art nursing center in Chelsea, Massachusetts. It was conceived to be a home rather than a hospital and to provide a greenhouse environment where each resident would receive individualized nursing care with all of the conveniences we expect in our day-to-day surroundings. It accepted people of varied levels of income and illness. It was built as an example of what is possible when a different approach and mindset is applied to providing long-term care. It was actually the first urban Green House in the United States.

There are ten condominium-style homes on six floors, each with its own front door and doorbell. Each home is 7,000 square feet and consists of ten private bedrooms that are arranged in suite fashion around a common living room with a hearth, dining area, and kitchen. The format goes a long way to promoting a sense of family and community. Indeed, meals are served family style around a large table in the dining area.

Residents have access to an area known as Main Street, designed to provide the stores and services one finds in a community (for example, a café, bakery, deli, chapel, and European day spa) and a community area where residents can meet and visit with friends, relatives, and fellow residents. Some of the amenities provided are similar to those found at a five-star resort.

The center provides services for both long-term care as well as short-term rehabilitation. A unique feature of the center is that it also provides housing for patients with Amyotrophic Lateral Sclerosis, known as ALS or Lou Gehrig's disease, and for Multiple Sclerosis (MS), who are not able to live independently. These high-tech rooms enable a person to maintain the highest level of independence. Since opening its doors in 2010, it has been recognized worldwide as an innovative model of care for senior citizens.

I visited the Leonard Florence Center for Living. It was a thriving, living example of what is possible. It was exactly as it is described—beautiful, warm, inviting. Each person I encountered who lived and worked there seemed happy and content. It was a truly memorable experience.

CHELSEA JEWISH NURSING HOME—Chelsea, Massachusetts

Chelsea Jewish Nursing Home, providing skilled nursing and rehabilitation, is the facility that inspired Barry Berman to build Leonard Florence Center for Living. It is a 120-bed facility, perched on a hill, surrounded by small houses and apartment buildings. This is the original building in which Barry Berman first placed his mother after she had her stroke. In a matter of only a few days, he was shocked and horrified by the change in his mother's demeanor and appearance. Thankfully, Barry Berman had the resources to take his mother home and provide the care and therapy she needed. However, from that point, he was not only on a mission to build a facility that embodies a different model of care, but also to transform Chelsea Jewish to emulate that model to the greatest extent possible.

I recently visited Chelsea Jewish and had the chance to meet with its executive director, Edward Stewart. I drove up the hill to a rather unassuming gray building and was lucky enough to find a parking spot across from the entrance on the somewhat narrow street. There were several steps leading up to the entrance, and an electronic sliding door that opened to a small lobby which reflected the small facility size. However, to the right of the reception desk was an inviting, bright dining and café area with large picture windows where residents, families, and visitors could relax while eating their meals or enjoying their visits. Coffee, tea, light beverages, bakery, and café fare are available at all times throughout the day at no cost.

I was particularly impressed that when I approached the reception desk and gave the young woman receptionist my first name, she had not only been informed of my appointment, but also the fact that I was running a few minutes late due to the traffic I encountered traveling from my previous appointment. She conveyed a warm, friendly, efficient manner that set the tone for everything I encountered during my visit.

Mr. Stewart, a seasoned professional who had been at the facility for four years, came to greet me within a few moments. After brief introductions, the conversation immediately turned to the facility and how it had been transformed.

The model is based on the Green House Project, and as such, the transformation involved reconstruction of the interior of the facility.

We proceeded to visit the upper long-term care areas—called "homes" rather than "units" (as they're typically referred to in a more institutional setting). Upon stepping off the elevator on the floor of the dementia care home I could see that it was vastly different from other such "units" in the typical institutional-type nursing home. The elevator doors opened to a fairly wide carpeted hallway that was comfortably lit and painted in soothing colors.

We entered what was essentially the common dining and sitting area. Staff members were seated next to residents, actively engaging with them in a variety of activities based on their level of ability. There was none of what one commonly sees: residents sitting idly and staring blankly into space, TV blaring with irrelevant programming, staff members sitting off to the side overseeing a group of people as if they were "babysitting" (for lack of a better word), ordering residents to sit down when they attempted to get up from their chairs, no one hustling back and forth in the hallways rushing to perform a variety of custodial tasks, no central nursing station with phones ringing, medical charts, or clanging bells.

There was a small office with an open door which constituted the space for the nurse on the floor, though that person was not sequestered at the desk doing work. Behind that office was a narrow hallway that led to a seating area with charts and computers where staff members could sit and complete their assigned desktop tasks. One nurse was dispensing medication from a somewhat typical-looking medication cart. Upon questioning, I learned that the medication cart was a remaining remnant of the former traditional environment and the facility was looking into purchasing something that resembled more of a piece of furniture. Overall, it was a calm, peaceful setting that evoked the feeling of a homelike living environment. It was unlike anything I had seen before. I felt that if I personally needed this kind of care, here I would be in a comfortable, dignified environment with a truly caring staff.

The central kitchen in the facility had been eliminated; this is considered essential for any transformation to a green house model. Each floor has two homes, which means there is a kitchen area for each. Cooks assigned to each kitchen prepare each of the three meals and are educated in the specific dietary and food consistency needs of each resident. The residents gather to eat with one another at a central table, and some areas contain a few smaller side tables that accommodate a smaller number of people.

What struck me as the most incredible were the staffing ratios. I was told that six certified nurse aides are assigned to forty residents on each floor. In addition, each unit has a homemaker. The homemaker is responsible for making beds, tidying and cleaning rooms, bathrooms and common areas, serving food, and cleaning up after meals. They also assist with delivering and hanging the laundered clothing.

The CNA tasks are strictly resident/patient-related: bathing, dressing, AM and PM routines, feeding, turning, positioning, and range of motion as needed, etc. This division of responsibility and staffing ratio allows for sufficient attention aimed at meeting the needs and providing the care that each resident requires without the typical stress, tension, and rush that most CNAs experience in more traditional models. In those settings, there may be as few as two aides on the lowest end of the spectrum (which I have unfortunately seen) to a maximum of five (though that is a rarer occurrence) assigned to forty residents. However, in the more traditional model, the CNA is not only responsible for the bathing, dressing, AM and PM care routines, feeding, and positioning, but also for making beds and tidying rooms. There is usually a central laundry responsible for washing and delivering clothing to resident rooms, (some facilities contract with an outside laundry service) and porters who are responsible for cleaning rooms, bathrooms, hallways, and common areas.

I asked Mr. Stewart how the facility is able to provide the high staffing ratios and continue to be financially solvent. His answer was astounding and refreshing. As an executive director—essentially the administrator—he does not have an executive assistant. I received the same answer from Barry Berman, the CEO of the organization. The salaries for administrative positions are saved by reducing salaries at the top levels in favor of spending on care for the residents. Those on the administrative level of the company share personnel as needed. There is a central admissions department, marketing department, accounting department, and so on.

Adding to the homelike environment is a European day spa. Here residents can receive traditional spa services (e.g., facials, massages) that can be scheduled by appointment but also provide a means of decreasing anxiety and agitation on an as-needed basis. The hair salon provides the typical services one would find in a community salon setting; manicures and pedicures are also available by appointment. These services are all included in the daily reimbursement room rate the facility receives.

Chelsea Jewish Nursing Home reflects what is possible when the right mindset is applied for providing a respectful, dignified, quality care environment for our elder citizens as they advance through the years of their lives.

NEW BRIDGE ON THE CHARLES—Boston, Massachusetts

New Bridge on the Charles is a retirement community in the suburbs of Boston.

It is built according to a traditional model and provides a continuum of care— independent living, assisted living, and a wing with nursing home beds. However, the section that houses the nursing home beds is structured very differently from the traditional sterile, institutional environments.

This facility was organized to resemble a household. Each of sixteen people have their own individual rooms built around a shared common living area, kitchen, and dining room. These living spaces are called "pods." The households are similar in size to many traditional living spaces in the community. Research has found that in units with less than twenty people, there tends to be less anxiety and depression, more socializing and friendship, an increased sense of safety, and more interaction with staff—even when patients have developed dementia.[72]

The staff at New Bridge have a different approach to their job. There are no traditional nursing stations. Instead they move among the residents and interact with them freely. An open-air design allows residents to view and interact with other members of their "pod household," creating more of a sense of community and sharing as they engage in familiar day-to-day activities. These include such simple but real-life activities as going to the kitchen to get a snack or watching other people have a friendly conversation, listening to music, or playing cards. In Atul Gawande's book *Being Mortal*, he reports how residents at New Bridge describe feeling as though they are living in a home. One resident in particular described being so much happier with her stay at New Bridge as compared to a more traditional facility, which she referred to as an "asylum."[73]

Another added benefit is that New Bridge shares its grounds with a private school, kindergarten through eighth grades. Louise Hay contends that it is important for us to have contact with all generations. Children's laughter in particular and connecting with children in general keeps us young at heart. Children are the foundation of life and future generations. Being around them often provides elder citizens with a vitality that comes from the joy of watching them move and play.[74]

At New Bridge, a program allows residents who are more capable to act as tutors to the young schoolchildren. This also creates important kinships, links with previous generations, and helps develop an appreciation of what an older person can provide in experience and wisdom—something lost but sorely needed in our society.

The children pay monthly visits to New Bridge, put on shows, and share holiday celebrations. When middle schoolers study World War II or other historical events, they are able to learn about them from the firsthand experiences of the residents who were veterans. Older children are also taught to understand and work with people who have dementia.

You might be thinking that New Bridge is a place for those with significant financial means. This is fortunately not the case. Many of the residents are just regular working people who had all but used up their savings and receive government assistance. The facility has prospered through the generosity of philanthropic financial donors.

PETER SANBORN PLACE—Reading, Massachusetts

Peter Sanborn Place was built in 1983. It is a seventy-three-unit apartment building intended for independent, low-income residents from the local community. As the residents aged in the community, the issue of how to care for them arose. The prospect of sending them to a traditional nursing home was viewed as unacceptable.

At first, residents needed help with simple day-to-day chores, such as shopping, laundry, and cleaning. The director at the time, Jacqueline Carson, arranged for agency aides to help as needed. However, as medical situations changed and needs progressed, there was a clear need for more specialized medical staff, such as physical therapists and nurses.

Eventually, there was an outcry from the local agencies who began to insist that the residents be sent to nursing homes. Ms. Carson objected. Rather than acquiesce, she formed her own agency, hiring her own workers, aides, and professionals to provide the services needed by the residents.

Ten years later, only thirteen of the seventy-three residents were independent; however, they all remained at Sanborn Place. Several of the residents with advanced dementia or Alzheimer's disease now require round the clock attention. Throughout the process, Ms. Carson was adamant that Sanborn Place remain known as an "apartment complex." Because of her steadfast commitment to this premise, it has avoided any reclassification as a nursing home or assisted living facility.

BEACON HILL VILLAGES—Boston, Massachusetts

Beacon Hill Villages is a community-based cooperative that offers assistance and service to elderly residents who remain in their homes. A grassroots nonprofit 501(C)(3) membership organization, it is funded through membership fees and private donations. The first village opened in 2002, and to date there are more than 140 such villages throughout the world. Each village offers a wide range of services that residents may need, such as plumbing, cleaning, shopping, and laundry.

Beacon Hill Village's premise is similar to those above—to offer people a sense of dignity and autonomy as they age. Their mantra is that they direct their own lives and create their own future. The adage "it takes a village to raise a child" seems to have been reinterpreted by Beacon Hill Villages: "It takes community to consider the needs of its elders and to provide what's needed to care for them."

ROCKPORT HEALTH CARE—Los Angeles, California

Rockport Healthcare Services has over seventy for-profit nursing home facilities under its umbrella. As of October 2018, when I spoke with Matthew Lysobey, the company's chief community integration officer, all of the facilities except one were located in California. The programs Matthew oversees in each of the facilities is nothing short of remarkable. This further underscores the point that with a modicum of creativity, the correct mindset and attitude toward those who, for whatever reason, must live in a nursing home, anything is possible. People need a purpose for living no matter what their age, and it can be found if one is dedicated to looking for ways to provide it.

This could not be better exemplified by two of the programs Matthew described.

The first one occurs in each of the seventy-plus facilities. Residents travel into the community to help prepare and serve food at local homeless shelters. There is no additional cost to the facility as it is considered part of the budget allocated for weekly activity outings; residents are transported by facility-owned vehicles. The cost of the food comes from the homeless shelter budget.

All residents are encouraged to participate, including those who have advancing Alzheimer's disease, Parkinson's disease, paralysis after a stroke, and so on. All members of the team work together to make it a rewarding experience for the residents, both psychosocially and physically. As Matthew explained it to me: "Even a person with advancing dementia can use a scoop to place salad, macaroni and cheese, etc., on to someone's plate." The person who is paralyzed or weak can use an adaptive device to complete a desired task. There are few circumstances that would preclude a person from participating. All those who have the desire do so; however, there are instances when tender encouragement is needed. It goes such a long way to having people feel useful; they are doing something to serve their community, to help others, and continue to feel they are relevant, contributing members of society. The sense of pleasure, belonging, thankfulness, and purpose exchanged between the person at the homeless shelter receiving the food and the resident from the facility serving the food is immeasurable. As Matthew explained, it's the love you put into it that is important. It is truly a "heart to serve" program. It is estimated that the total meals served by Rockport Healthcare services is between five thousand and six thousand a month.

The second program he described is a senior canine adoption program, which the facility runs in cooperation with local animal shelters. Dogs are assessed for eligibility and compatibility with the nursing home environment. Trainers from the animal shelter assess and train residents in appropriate animal care.

The purpose of the program is for the nursing home to nurture senior dogs that would otherwise be "put down" at local shelters. Residents are assigned tasks based on their level of ability: brushing, filling feeding bowls, walking, playing, ensuring safe and secure placement at night, etc. A facility resident is selected as a foster dog volunteer for the shelter. This person is essentially the go-to person when the pet is ready for adoption. As information is disseminated to the community about seeking a home for a particular animal, the designated resident representative for the facility obtains the pertinent information and the residents vote on the appropriateness of a particular placement. This goes way beyond the notion of a visiting pet therapy program.

Once again, with the right attitude, mindset, and a healthy dose of creativity, the path to providing a dignified, respectful living environment that affords each person a sense of belonging and purpose is attainable.

ASSOCIATION MONTESSORI INTERNATIONAL (AMI)

Maria Montessori developed a philosophy of child-centered education in which the education curriculum is essentially guided by the child's interest level and abilities. There are many Montessori schools around the world. My own children attended a Montessori preschool, and my daughter continued to attend through first grade.

The philosophy of child-centered education has recently been extended to a person-centered approach to caring for our elder citizens and is particularly applicable to those afflicted with Alzheimer's and dementia. As the disease progresses, those individuals may not be able to verbally express their interests or abilities, just as young children may not. However, the astute observer can design the environment geared toward the needs, strengths, and abilities of individuals.

In 2014, Association Montessori International created a Montessori Advisory Group to developing a Montessori Approach for Dementia and Aging. The approach encourages a person to function at their highest ability throughout the entire course of their lives. It provides an adaptive environment that supports the individual through the stages of memory loss as well as a sensory environment to facilitate and maintain independence at the highest possible level. This "prepared" environment as envisioned by Dr. Montessori provides opportunities for freedom of movement, is structured and orderly, has easy access to nature, is beautiful, and provides specialized materials that meet individuals' cognitive needs.[75]

The environment would place carefully planned memory, visual, auditory, tactile, and olfactory cues throughout the environment with the necessary cues required to capture the individual's attention. As Alzheimer's disease and associated dementia progress, the person declines in their ability to recognize or negotiate objects in the environment. Therefore, needed signs on the walls in the environment should be painted with bright or contrasting colors to capture a person's visual attention.

In addition, individuals would have the opportunity to participate in familiar routines that could provide meaning to their lives such as cleaning, washing, or dusting. There would be outdoor gardens that would encourage planting, weeding, or raking as needed. The materials needed to complete any of these tasks would be clearly visible in a safe fashion so they could be accessed as the individual's need or desire arises.

I would also advocate the use of brightly colored dishes to capture and maintain attention during mealtime and ensure that colors of the food on the plate are also of differing colors. We all eat with our eyes first, as evidenced by TV commercials and advertisements with pictures of juicy, colorful food that capture our attention and get our mouths watering. All too often the plates, utensils, and food in facilities are pale in color and basically blend into one another. When this is combined with a declining ability to maintain attention to tasks, including the task of eating, it could result in a reduced ability to identify the food on the plate and a loss of interest in eating entirely. Brightly colored food, plates, and utensils could make an important difference.

Furthermore, consistent with the Montessori philosophy, an individual would be able to continue caring for him or herself (e.g., bathing, dressing) as long as possible. This is the very essence of independence and goes a long way to promote self-respect and dignity. Individuals are also encouraged to help one another as long as they are safe and capable of doing so. The concept of helping others is known to promote meaningful relationships, increases a sense of purpose, and contributes to an individual's sense of well-being and self-esteem.

There is strong evidence-based information that for those individuals who participate in the "Montessori for Dementia and Aging" approach, there is a significant reduction in antipsychotic and sedative medication drug use. This reduction was maintained in an eighteen-month follow-up study.[76] Fewer feeding difficulties were noted, and individuals demonstrated improved ability to feed themselves independently for a longer period of time.[77] Communication interactions also improved.

I found it interesting that the environment described in the Montessori approach is similar to one that I suggested to the administration of a facility in a section of my previous book *Nursing Home to Rehabilitation Centers: What Every Person Needs to Know*. Though I have seen facilities attempt to incorporate some of these concepts, they have been feeble at best and did not demonstrate an understanding or true commitment to the concept, which also requires intensive staff training.

The environment proposed in the "Montessori for Dementia and Aging" approach is not dissimilar to the environment we create for children from their early stages of infancy to early childhood. The progression of disease amounts to a regression of sorts. However, one must always remember that individuals with Alzheimer's disease and dementia are not children, but adults who have lived a life of experiences and varied levels of knowledge. Shouldn't we, therefore, be providing a safe, caring, nurturing environment for these elders as we would for our children?

Obstacles in Positively Transforming
Traditional Nursing Homes

Considering research dating back to the early 1970s and the growth of alternative models for eldercare, all of which validate the fact that individuals do better medically, physically, and emotionally, why has there not been a significant change in how we care for our elder citizens?

Why have the more traditional models continued to grow and thrive? Why have lawmakers not done more to ensure better environments and ultimately better care for our elder citizens?

One major drawback to the alternative models, especially the Green House Project, is the limited numbers of elder citizens they can accommodate—ten to twelve elders per home environment or "pod." The vast numbers of the ever-growing aging population, as well as those with Alzheimer's disease or dementia that may need care outside of the family home will unfortunately dictate to some extent facility size and design.

A traditional nursing home typically has over a hundred beds, with many upwards of two hundred. Furthermore, although there are some private rooms in nursing homes, most have two beds, some three or four. The idea is to maximize the number of beds to maximize the income.

There is an inverse relationship between the number of beds and staffing. The idea is to provide the minimal staffing possible to maximize profit. In the Green House homes, the focus is on improved quality of life. That is not to say the homes are not profitable, but this consideration does not supercede quality of life and quality of care.

The cost of building these facilities per bed significantly outweighs the cost for traditional nursing homes; however, the costs are mainly related to construction. In some ways, because of the different way the homes are organized, the operational costs can be less. There is no central kitchen because each home has its own kitchen. This eliminates the personnel costs of a dietary department, including kitchen workers who are involved with food preparation, service, and cleanup.

Because the homes have private bathrooms, there is no patient-to-patient contact. Therefore, some of the costs related to infection control may be reduced or eliminated.

Limited elements of the "alternative philosophy" have crept into the traditional nursing home model. These changes have been incorporated, often in some perverted way, because they were practically thrust upon the industry by others with only limited understanding of the "new trends" based on these alternative models. However, because they are introduced in a limited way and superimposed on top of the traditional styles of nursing home care, functionally they are little more than window dressing. All too often people still sit, staring vacantly at TV screens or sensory stimulation sporadically placed on the walls. Pleasant things to see and hear are not near patient areas but found in hallways. Patients who can barely walk are unable to see them.

Current nursing industry attempts may include renaming units with cute colloquial names and referring to them as "communities" or "neighborhoods." "Pet therapy" is often reduced to someone coming to the facility once or twice a week with a couple of dogs, visiting the units and allowing individuals to pet the animals for a few minutes. Some facilities have birds in the reception areas as well as in cages in or near a recreational room or rehabilitation department. You might see someone sitting and looking at them from time to time, but they offer little beyond that. The most out-of-the-box idea of "pet therapy" I saw in the traditional model was a facility that brought in a pony once a week.

The Department of Health survey process has now changed to be more "resident-centered," but unless substantial changes are made to the living environments, it has the potential to amount to little more than a buzzword. The quality of life, quality of care, staffing levels, overall environment, routines, and general functioning of the facility for the most part is still unchanged from the traditional model. Therefore, the experience for the long-term care resident or short-term rehabilitation patient remains essentially the same.

One facility spent thousands of dollars to install a huge fish tank in the lobby. The stated purpose was so residents could sit and look at it and it would also "look good" when people entered the building. This is a far cry from Bill Thomas' concept at Chase Memorial.

Traditional nursing homes also operate as medical models under strict guidelines from the Centers of Medicare and Medicaid Services as well as each state's Department of Health. The facilities' primary focus is to comply with those regulations. Interviews with nurse aides reveal that the emphasis on routines and care schedules as well as that of safety in the traditional long-term care makes it difficult for staff to provide residents with choice and self-determination.[78]

In order to transform these facilities, a close examination and redesign of the guidelines would be required by these regulatory bodies in order to adapt a more psychosocial model in which the real needs of the individual would be the top priority.

It took visionaries like Keren Brown Wilson, Bill Thomas, Barry Berman, and Jacqueline Carson who were dedicated to providing an improved quality of care and quality of life. If one cares and provides what is needed to promote that, profit will follow. It takes loud, persistent voices to make those changes happen.

Everyday Remedies

A facility should function in a way that the individual can continue to feel comfortable and familiar. A prime example would be an individual with a common cold or cough. Many of us have treated these simple ailments throughout our lifetime with everyday remedies: increasing the amount and frequency of liquids such as hot tea, soup, and juices, especially those containing vitamin C, and sucking on cough drops. A study back in October 2000 by the American College Of Chest Physicians supported chicken soup as a cold remedy.[79] Yet I have seen little or none of this in any of the over forty facilities in which I have worked. The common "tried and true" treatment is a prescription for Robitussin.

But why not incorporate these home remedies into the regimen in the long-term care environment? Is it because the medical model is so inextricably linked to the pharmaceutical industry? Even under the present medical model, couldn't a doctor prescribe frequent juices, hot tea, or soup to a resident with a common cold or cough? How many among us have gone to a doctor with those ailments, or even with a mild flu, only to have the doctor prescribe bed rest and those very same remedies? Other cultures may have other remedies for these common ailments that are equally successful.

Holistic Considerations

In being committed to viewing the person as a "whole" in terms of mind, body, and spirit, new techniques could be incorporated that have been well documented as contributing to an individual's overall health and wellness, especially when combined with traditional medical techniques. These have come to be known as holistic or homeopathic remedies.

Some hospitals have begun incorporating these modalities into their paradigm of care, recognizing the positive effect they have in helping patients not only cope with their illness but also become active participants in the healing process. These patients also may become more compliant with traditional medical treatments. In particular, patients experiencing anxiety, depression, or pain can benefit from this approach on an individual or small group basis.

Among the holistic modalities that have been successfully incorporated into hospital settings are acupuncture, aromatherapy, guided imagery, healing touch, massage, meditation, relaxation, and yoga. These modalities should be provided by licensed health care professionals who have received advanced education and training in integrative health and holistic healing. Yoga in particular is having widespread use in a patient's ability to cope with pain and is being used to wean patients off opioids and other strong pain medication.[80]

Some facilities attempt to incorporate some of these modalities by introducing activities such as tai chi on a monthly or bimonthly basis. However, these "activities" are usually presented to large groups for only thirty or sixty minutes. This is due in part because these activities are necessary for the facility to provide, but they are not necessarily ones that generate revenue or contribute to reimbursement in a significant way. This does not constitute a legitimate attempt to provide alternative techniques from which the resident could derive maximum benefit. For that to occur, the modality would have to be provided much as other ancillary therapy services are provided—individually on at least a weekly or biweekly basis.

As stated in previous chapters, the present system functions in a way that is all too easy for owners to find loopholes to maximize profit. In this system, profit is the primary motivation for the owners. The nursing homes that have any desire to transform their facility to resemble anything remotely related to a Green House would have to have a fundamental commitment to the notion that skilled nursing facilities could provide care to our elder citizens in a vastly different way than they do presently. Concomitantly, the regulatory bodies that oversee facilities would have to set a course which acknowledges and addresses these alternative approaches.

Is it practical to think that a sufficient number of new homes can be built in the style of the Green House Project to accommodate our ever-growing elder population? Probably not.

However, can we examine the over 15,000 existing nursing homes and insist that they be transformed to provide improved dignity, respect, quality of life, and quality of care for our elder citizens? If the priorities and the mindset truly change, we certainly can make progress toward improving how care in nursing homes is delivered.

What will it take for this change to occur?

One of the ways is for the "bean counters" to be removed from the equation as an important voice in nursing home design and operations. Will that be a decision they make independently? Will they agree to it without a fight? I'm sure we all would agree that will not be the case. What will it take for them to realize that they can continue to be financially successful while at the same time providing quality care, a dignified and respectful LIVING environment, placing emphasis on individual's needs and developing competent, compassionate empathetic staff?

Can we leave it solely to advocacy organizations such as National Consumer Voice for Quality Long Term Care, the Long-Term Care Community Coalition, Consumer Watch,or regulatory bodies such as Center for Medicare Advocacy? Can we rely on the many articles written by journalists, researchers and pundits that have appeared in newspapers around the country that highlight the many issues described in this book?

Who will replace them?

It will take a loud and persistent outcry from the population at large. *Conversation is necessary to effect change.* Therefore, it is up to *us*—each one of us. *We* each need to be part of the conversation, boldly insisting on a change in the attitudes and culture of care for our parents, our elder citizens, our loved ones.

EIGHT

ALZHEIMER'S DISEASE AND DEMENTIA —A GROWING ISSUE FOR US ALL

Examples of Inappropriate Use of Medication to Control Behavior

I had been asked to evaluate a resident who was having difficulty swallowing. I was only told that she ate in her room and was receiving puree consistency. As it was shortly before the noon meal, I had to go directly to her room before checking any other chart information. I entered after knocking on the opened door. When I approached her bed, which was on the far side of the room next to the window, I found a rather frail, gaunt woman approximately in her mid-eighties laying completely flat in her bed. I was unnerved to see the position of the bed and how it was affecting her. Not only did she look extremely uncomfortable, but the position also was unsafe. Her head was tilted backward against the bed, and this caused her mouth to be wide open; it was obviously dry from breathing. She was wearing a pretty flowered dress, although it seemed too large for her tiny frame. There were no teeth in her mouth. She was not asleep, but she was not fully alert either; she certainly would not have been able to operate the bed's remote control to put herself in that position.

I bent over to gently say hello so I could make eye contact with her and explain the purpose of my visit. At that moment, a male nurse entered the room through the open door and approached the resident's bed. He was holding a small medication cup in hand one hand and a small white plastic spoon in the other. The applesauce in the cup obviously contained medication that had been crushed.

He spoke with a pronounced accent. He said what was intended for the resident, but he didn't talk directly to her. He seemed to be "talking to the air" as he said he was going to give her medication. Simultaneously, in one swift motion he dug the spoon into the small cup, loaded it with medication-laced applesauce, and attempted to put the spoon into her mouth while she was laying completely flat. This all happened so swiftly, that I didn't have the chance to say anything. Of course, the resident was totally confused, taken by surprise, and probably afraid. She immediately picked up her hand and swatted at the nurse's hand with the spoon that contained the applesauce. The applesauce went flying off the spoon onto the bedsheet. The nurse exclaimed, "Oh no!"

At the same moment, I blurted out, "You can't do that. You can't give someone medication laying completely flat—she could choke."

I concentrated on comforting the resident. I leaned over and looked her in the eyes once again and gently touched her shoulder. I assured her that no one wanted to hurt her and explained I was going to gently raise the head of the bed so she could sit up and take her medication before eating her lunch. I pushed the button on the bed remote, raising the head of the bed in small amounts, very slowly. Finally, the head of the bed reached the upright position. I told the nurse I would give her the remainder of the medication. He gave me the small plastic cup with the applesauce and the small white plastic spoon. He remained in the room and looked on.

I looked the patient in the eyes, stroked her shoulder and gently told her I would be giving her the medication. I showed her the spoon, inserted it into the plastic cup and put a small amount on the spoon. She willingly opened her mouth and took the medication. I did this repeatedly about three or four times until she had taken all of the medication that remained in the small plastic cup. She seemed comfortable and relaxed. I told her I would have someone come to bring her lunch, and I left the room with the nurse.

Once I left the room, I reported the incident to the nurse manager sitting at the nurse's station. She said she would educate the nurse about proper positioning for giving patients medication.

<hr/>

Of course, the positioning was extremely important, but I told her it was equally important to educate the nurse about how to approach patients, especially those who were confused. I explained what could have possibly happened if I wasn't in the room:

> The nurse would have reported that the patient was refusing to take her medication—that she tried to hit him while he was trying to give it to her. When she swatted at his hand much of the medication fell onto her bedsheet. He would *not* have reported that the patient was lying flat, or that he merely tried pushing the spoon in her mouth loaded with applesauce without even looking at her or trying to get her attention. The situation then could have been reported to the doctor as follows: the resident refused to take her medication, she was "acting out," and attempted to hit the nurse. As a result, the doctor may have prescribed an antipsychotic medication for the patient. While this would have been an entirely inappropriate use of antipsychotic medication, unfortunately this is not an atypical example. How could this have affected the resident? She could have become lethargic and less able to adequately respond to, or interact, with her environment.

E.H., a fairly alert and verbal patient in her early seventies was admitted to a short-term rehabilitation unit after being hospitalized for the repair of a broken hip. She had signs of early onset dementia; she was mildly, albeit pleasantly confused. On this particular morning E.H. had to use the bathroom before she began eating her breakfast, which had already been delivered to her room, located just a few doors down from the nursing station. She rang for assistance, but after almost three-quarters of an hour, no one came to assist her with her toileting needs.

In a desperate attempt to get someone's attention, she picked up the tray from the bedside table, and with all her might, she flung it into the doorway directly across from her bed. This, of course, had the desired effect; nurses and nurse aides came running to the room to find out what had happened. The patient explained that she had been ringing for assistance to use the bathroom and no one had come to assist her. She feared having an "accident" in the bed (obviously a degrading and humiliating experience); her solution was to make as much noise as possible to get the immediate attention she needed.

Staff follow-up to the incident concluded that the "behavior" presented by E. H. needed to be addressed. The physician obliged by prescribing antipsychotic medications that would have a calming effect to prevent further "acting-out" behaviors.

When the family came to visit their mother the following day, they were outraged when they learned what had transpired. They objected vehemently to the antipsychotic medication that was prescribed. They insisted that their mother never had any "behavioral issues" and her actions were the direct result of the reduced response time of the nursing staff to attend to her immediate biological needs. They threatened to call the appropriate state agencies to report the matter. Needless to say, the prescribed medications were immediately discontinued.

Mr. F.S. was a Spanish-speaking gentleman who had been living with his daughter. All members of the family worked during the day, and he was no longer able to safely stay alone. His judgment was now impaired: he was unable to take his medication, safely use the stove, or adequately prepare something to eat. There had been a few instances of him walking out of the apartment and wandering aimlessly into the neighborhood. His daughter feared for his safety and her family's meager resources did not allow her to provide adequate care for him during the long hours that the family was out of the home. Ultimately, she felt she had no choice but to admit him to the long-term care unit of a skilled nursing facility. Mr. F.S. seemed saddened by being away from his family, and the situation was made somewhat worse by the fact that few people in these new, unfamiliar surroundings spoke his language.

The morning of the second day after his admission, the nurse aide assigned to him for the day entered his room to wake him for breakfast. She was from a different culture, with a thick accent and a rough, brisk demeanor. In her loud, no-nonsense style, she informed Mr. F.S. that it was time for him to get up and eat breakfast. He was still in bed and half-asleep. Though I wasn't there when the incident occurred, I can envision what may have happened.

Mr. F.S. opened his eyes to see a strange person with a loud voice looming over him while he lay in bed. The surroundings were still unfamiliar, and he did not understand the words the person was saying. He was probably fearful and may have interpreted that the stranger in his room was there to cause him harm. He lashed out and attempted to hit the aide. She ran out of the room and called the nurse. The nurse, from a different culture than both the resident and the nurse aide, spoke English with a decided accent. She accompanied the aide to the room and tried to subdue the resident to no avail. Their next course of action: call 911. The police came and removed the resident from the facility. He returned a few hours later. The incident was reported to the physician who prescribed an antipsychotic medication to "control" his behavior. The family was informed that their father began to act out and hit the staff. They were informed of the drugs that were prescribed, but it is uncertain if a full explanation of the drugs or their side effects were explained or understood. The result was that Mr. F.S. became completely lethargic. Thereafter, he had difficulty holding his utensils to feed himself and he was much less alert. He had a faraway look in his eyes and when he was spoken to, his responses were slow, his voice was very soft, almost inaudible, and his speech was slurred.

The use of antipsychotic medications as a method of "controlling" behavior is a serious concern for the residents in our nation's nursing homes, and even more for those with Alzheimer's disease or dementia. A 2015 federal report by the Government Accountability Office revealed that an average of approximately 30 percent of all elder residents with a diagnosis of dementia residing in nursing homes received antipsychotic drugs at some point during their stay. Short-term-stay patients were prescribed antipsychotic medications 23 percent of the time compared with 33 percent for residents in a long-term stay.[81] According to a GAO report earlier that same year, one in three nursing home residents were at risk for being prescribed these dangerous drugs.[82] In December 2018, National Public Radio reported that nearly one in five nursing home residents were taking dangerous antipsychotic drugs. A report from the Government Accountability Office and AARP Public Policy Institute finds that antipsychotic drugs are now also overprescribed for dementia patients who are living at home or in assisted living facilities, estimated to be one in seven individuals.[83] It should be known that antipsychotic drugs are not approved by the Federal Drug Administration for treatment of dementia; they are restricted for cases of serious mental illnesses (i.e., schizophrenia, bipolar disorder). The warning on the boxes of these medications are known as a "black box warning" and indicate that when prescribed for elder patients with dementia, they can increase the risk of death.[84] What are the side effects of these dangerous medications? They result in an individual appearing to be dull and lethargic with reduced ability to interact, respond, express their needs and wants, and as a result are at an increased risk for falling.

In February 2015, an article entitled "'They Want Docile': How Nursing Homes in the United States Overmedicate Patients with Dementia" was issued by Human Rights Watch.[85] The summary of the article quotes Walter L, an eighty-one-year-old gentleman who was a resident in a Texas facility in December 2016. He described the situation as follows:

> Too many times I'm given too many pills. . . . [Until they wear off,] I can't even talk. I have a thick tongue when they do that. I ask them not to [give me the antipsychotic drugs]. When I say that, they threaten to remove me from the [nursing] home. They get me so I can't think. I don't want anything to make me change the person I am.

In the same summary, a director of nursing in a facility in Kansas described what her facility was like prior to reducing the use of antipsychotic medications by 50 percent in January 2017.

> It used to be like a death prison here. We cut our antipsychotics in half in six months. Half our residents were on antipsychotics. Only 10 percent of our residents have a mental illness.

This is not only a serious issue for dementia patients in and out of our nursing home facilities, it is considered an international human rights violation to administer antipsychotic medications to control people against their will or knowledge in any situation that is not of an emergency nature. Yet obtaining consent from a person with dementia, especially one that is elderly, can be extremely difficult. According to the article, Human Rights Watch was able to determine that in many cases "nursing facilities made no effort to obtain meaningful, informed consent from the individual or a health proxy before administering the medications in cases where it clearly would have been possible to do so."[86]

To date, 20 percent of the individuals in nursing homes—approximately 250,000 frail, elderly, infirm people—continue to receive these powerful drugs, and only 2 percent of them have a diagnosis that would warrant prescriptions for these medications. Furthermore, despite the fact that the Centers for Medicare and Medicaid Services has added protocols to their survey process for the Department of Health in each state,, to identify and determine the situations in which antipsychotic medications are inappropriately prescribed and to issue citations accordingly, 99.5 percent of the time, the finding has been that there was no actual harm to the resident. There must be more effective, less harmful ways of caring for people experiencing mood swings or presenting with behavioral issues as a result of their changing cognitive status. But many of these issues are not necessarily related to cognition. As with the examples above, they may be due to staffing issues, language barriers, cultural diversity, lack of training, and the inability to approach and care for people in an empathetic manner.

As Alzheimer's disease progresses, the individual's ability to communicate and interact with others decreases; they seem to be withdrawing from the world and retreating further into themselves. In the final stages, the individual's abilities and behavior regress as follows: they may be unable to speak, unable to walk, unable to feed themselves or eat solid food. However, it should always be remembered that these are adults, each with a full life of experiences, likes and dislikes, preferences and opinions. If we think of this level of functioning as analogous to a that of a child as he or she develops, we can also see the difference in our responses to the child at this stage.

Many individuals, even in the advanced stages of the disease, remember on some deep-seated level the jobs and functions they had in their lives. I remember one resident who had worked in construction most of his life. As he walked from place to place, he would stop and look at the tiles on the floor and the wallpaper on the walls as if he were examining them to see if the work had been done satisfactorily. He would mumble and point to different spots as though he were telling someone the work was not done quite right. The staff recognized this as being important to him and never discouraged this behavior.

The difference with our response to children is that we look them in the eyes, smile at them, hug them, and engage with them in an effort to help them grow, learn to communicate, and learn to love. We engage in these behaviors lovingly, and in turn, an infant responds by looking at us, smiling or laughing, cooing and reaching out to touch us. But as the person with Alzheimer's disease retreats further away from the ability to communicate and engage with people, people tend to retreat from them as well. They are not acknowledged, people do not look them in their eyes or attempt to engage with them, and this ultimately deprives them of the love and affection we all need. All too often they are treated merely as bodies; people talk around them and do not relate to them as individuals in any way.

This reminds me of stories I've read about people who heard everything going on around them despite labeled as being in "a coma" or "a persistent vegetative state." If this is true in those situations, isn't it true for those individuals with Alzheimer's disease or dementia? Aren't they owed the same respect and dignity? Who is to say they aren't watching, seeing, and listening to everything going on around them and everything being said?[87] The importance of communication, compassion, empathy, and human touch cannot be overstated. AIDS patients in the early days of the disease have described their feelings of being deprived of human touch. There are studies that support the positive effects of human touch on the immune system, which in turn can increase serotonin, an important chemical in the human body. It is thought to affect the body's natural ability for maintaining a balanced mood and may have a "positive effect on social behavior, appetite, digestion, sleep and memory."[88] Conversely, low serotonin levels have been linked to depression and inflammation, which can place an individual at an increased risk for heart disease, arthritis, Type 2 diabetes, dementia, and even suicide.

An article in the Public Health Section of the *New York Times* reported that "older people who reported they felt left out, isolated or lacked companionship" decreased in their ability to perform daily activities: bathing, grooming, and preparing meals.[89] These feelings are rooted in the loneliness and boredom that many individuals in nursing homes experience. Therefore, owners need to take notice and design, or redesign, their facilities with programs to address these issues rather than utilizing drugs to address them.

LACK OF EMPATHY FOR ALZHEIMER'S OR DEMENTIA PATIENTS

One of the most virulent statements I have ever heard was made by a director of nursing, which made it that much more incredulous. It was said in the presence of a nurse manager staff member with whom I had worked several years prior at another facility. I have repeated this story many times, and each time I do, the person listening gasps in disbelief and then usually says that this person has no business being in the field of nursing. I told the administrator of the facility that I would share this story as one of the most egregious examples of lack of caring I have experienced in my career, and that I would repeat it because it was said directly to me—it is not gossip. It is an extreme example of what is wrong with the system and the potential for that system to take a turn in a disturbing direction.

I had been told that Medicare had become much more restrictive regarding the type and amount of food a person can eat by mouth if they are also receiving tube feeding. I was told that my patient would not be allowed to have more than a few sips of liquid or a few spoonfuls of pureed dessert (e.g., applesauce) and that if I prescribed more than that, the facility would not be reimbursed for the tube feeding. I couldn't believe my ears. I considered this beyond the pale of human decency.

Dementia or Alzheimer's patients may begin to eat and drink less as the disease progresses, which means they are not be able to eat sufficient amounts of food to sustain themselves. Often tube feeding supplements what the person eats by mouth to ensure their continued nutritional health. For example, someone might be able to eat a small amount of eggs in the morning, take bites of half a sandwich at noon, and maybe have a dessert snack and a small amount of food at dinner. Obviously this is not enough food for an older person to maintain their weight and stave off a variety of conditions. Though the individual may be eating, they may also be very confused and not aware of their surroundings or their place in them. Nevertheless, the person's swallowing ability may be sufficient for them to safely consume small amounts of solids and liquids.

There was extended conversation in this building about the facility losing money because of the lack of reimbursement for half a dozen patients who were eating consistencies other than puree, despite the fact that it did not amount to more than a small amount of food or liquid.

On this particular day, I was seated in the small office of the nurse manager discussing some of the residents on her unit who fell into this category. The director of nursing, a large woman, entered the cramped space and sat down to join the conversation. After hearing us discuss a few of the residents, she uttered these words: "If a person is that demented and doesn't know where they are, I don't know why we have to feed them anyway."

I was stunned and rendered almost speechless.

At that moment, all I could think of to say was that it was a quality of life issue and the Department of Health would certainly frown on that. I guess the statement I made instilled a sense of alarm and was interpreted to mean I would certainly consider making a phone call to the Department of Health to report the matter. Actually, I was only making what I considered to be an obvious statement and was too shocked to think of anything beyond how utterly flabbergasted I was to hear her say such a thing.

I reported it to the administrator, explaining how this attitude could impact the attitude of nurses toward residents in the facility, ultimately affecting their care.

Within a few days, the assistant administrator informed me that whether or not the facility received reimbursement for those residents receiving tube feeding who could also continue to eat, they would continue to provide whatever consistency or amount of food was appropriate. The director of nursing reversed what she had previously said to me to agree with the statement made by the assistant administrator.

———— ∞∞∞ ————

The impact something like this can have extends beyond patients with Alzheimer's disease or dementia. Most facilities would not want to accept a lack of reimbursement for a legitimate and needed medical intervention they are providing. This makes perfect sense. However, this can set a dangerous precedent. The impact could very likely be to pressure speech pathologists or other staff members not to feed or offer food to residents once they receive tube feeding.

Owners should be reimbursed for providing tube feeding, or any other legitimate service or treatment, if that is what the resident truly needs. It goes without saying that feeding, in whatever form it is provided, is essential to survival. I can't imagine why the consistency of the food a person is able to eat or drink is a determining factor in whether or not a facility receives reimbursement for tube feeding. As long as the person is unable to sustain themselves with food by mouth, and the medical need for the feeding tube has been established, than the reimbursement should be provided.

It is not unrealistic to think that there may be situations in which the decision will be made to withhold food from patients receiving tube feeding rather than fight with Medicare or lose money. What does that say about us as a society? If tube feeding is a medical intervention that is available and continues to be recommended based on an individual's medical condition, one thing should not preclude the other. Will patients or their families begin to be advised against tube feeding due to concern about lack of reimbursement despite the fact that patients cannot sustain themselves through eating by mouth? It is an example in the most severe forms of what is wrong with the system and the potential for it to take a disturbing downward spiral.

The Difference Between Alzheimer's Disease and Dementia

Alzheimer's disease and *dementia* are terms that are often used interchangeably; however, they have slightly different meanings.

Dementia is actually the result of changes that occur in the brain. The word is used to describe a series of brain disorders that cause a change or loss in ability to function in a variety of areas from thinking to social skills. The areas known as cognitive thinking or cognition include memory, orientation, attention, judgment, language and problem solving, and reasoning ability. Other areas of functioning that may be impacted are the ability to complete community-based tasks, home and hobbies, and personal care (also known as activities of daily living).

Dementia is usually diagnosed in stages ranging from no dementia to early stage, mid-stage, and finally late-stage. These stages tell us about the progression of the symptoms the person is experiencing. Each of these stages has a level of cognition that goes along with it that also gives us insight into the person's ability to function.[90]

Stage 1 – No cognitive decline

Stage 2 – Very mild. This comes across as normal forgetfulness. Many of us may experience this as we get older. That is not to say that all of us who experience this "normal forgetfulness" would be diagnosed with dementia; thus, the term *age associated memory impairment* is also used.

Stage 3 – Mild cognitive impairment. This stage may last a long time—sometimes even up to seven years—before any formal onset of dementia is diagnosed. At this stage, a person's family and friends may begin to notice signs or changes in the person's way of functioning.

Stage 4 – Moderate cognitive decline. This is usually when the term *mild dementia* is first applied. The person's difficulties become more pronounced at this stage. The person may actually recognize the difficulties but may also continue to deny them. As a result, they may tend to withdraw from social and family interactions.

Stage 5 – Moderate-severe cognitive decline. This is the beginning of the mid-stage. The person experiences major problems in independently completing personal care and activities of daily living and requires some assistance.

Stage 6 – Moderate-severe dementia. The person at this level requires considerable assistance.

Stage 7 – Very severe cognitive decline. This stage is associated with late-stage or severe dementia.

Alzheimer's disease, on the other hand, is actually that—a disease that results in dementia and is probably most commonly identified as being associated with it. There are other diseases that result in dementia and are progressive, which means they advance over time, and to date, are irreversible. The stages of the dementia associated with these other diseases may not follow the same course of the stages described above and may also have different components of dementia associated with them. Some of these may sound familiar: vascular dementia, Lewy body dementia, Parkinson's disease. Other changes to the brain may result in dementia but are not necessarily considered a disease per se. These include chronic alcohol or drug abuse, brain tumors, and traumatic brain injury.

One major area of functioning which is impacted by Alzheimer's disease is communication, which is also closely tied to the person's ability to remember. It stands to reason that if one cannot remember what they want to say, this will affect their ability to say it. We all experience this from time to time when we are trying to remember something and say, "It's on the tip of my tongue." Most of us eventually remember what we were trying to say: a word, a person's name, or a place. But the person with Alzheimer's disease has lost all recollection and cannot think of that word—not now, not later. It's like they have lost the use of their "Google" search engine.

There are different kinds of memory. One is the memory of how things are done, known as procedural memory. These include automatic tasks we do every day, such as brushing our teeth, combing our hair, or getting dressed. It also covers learned behaviors that we do repeatedly over time until they become automatic—how to drive a car, for example. Procedural memory is linked to more automatic behavior; it is more enduring.

The second type of memory is related to the knowledge of facts and information. Loss of memory in this area can be personal and functional, such as the names of family members or places, but it also includes less personally relevant information that is stored in our memory banks. Oftentimes short-term memory becomes more fleeting than long-term memory. In the case of the short-term memory loss, a person with Alzheimer's disease asks the same question over and over again. A strategy to counteract this might be writing down relevant information that person needs to remember and having it readily handy so they can refer to it when need be. It may help them feel more comfortable, confident, and more secure to know that when they are forgetful they can turn to something to help them recall.

But as the "words fail the person," they also can become easily frustrated, even angry. Though it is no fault of their own, it may even be hard for them to comprehend or accept the reasons that this is happening. Though it is intellectually understandable, it is often a difficult experience when interacting with the person who is behaving in that manner. Changes in the brain can affect changes in personality that may be difficult for family and loved ones. The individual may become angry and say things that were not typical of their behavior before the onset of the disease. It is all too easy to perceive oneself as being on the receiving end of that behavior, sometimes to even take it personally. However, this may not be the case.

Communication in all forms is an important ingredient in every person-to-person interaction, both verbal and nonverbal. Verbal generally refers to the words we use when speaking, but it may incorporate other elements such as tone of voice, the loudness and softness of the voice, and melody or intonation of the voice. Nonverbal communication generally refers to facial expression and gestures but may also incorporate environmental factors that may affect the message (e.g., background noise, visual distractions, crowded or roomy surroundings) Therefore, it goes without saying that is it important to consider both verbal and nonverbal factors when communicating with the individual who has Alzheimer's disease or dementia, not only because of the gaps they may be experiencing in their ability to recall and use words, but also because they may be conveying information nonverbally which the keen observer can detect and interpret to understand their intended meaning. Conversely, the individual with Alzheimer's disease or dementia may be more likely affected by nonverbal cues, especially as their ability to understand verbal language becomes more difficult. Therefore, when communicating with a person with dementia or Alzheimer's disease, the speaker should be aware of their own facial expression, volume and tone of their voice, gestures they are using, and any other signals, including environmental factors, that may be open to interpretation or misinterpretation. In addition, establishing eye contact and a gentle touch can go a long way in helping the person who is confused to feel calm, more secure, and more cared about. These are key elements of empathy and should be practiced by all staff members and caregivers who work in skilled nursing or assisted living facilities. They are especially important when working with individuals affected by Alzheimer's disease or dementia.

A wonderful program, "Music and Memory," has demonstrated the ability to improve communication with persons experiencing varying levels of cognitive impairment, as well as for people who are physically impaired. It was developed based on neuroscientific research by a social worker named Dan Cohen. The program creates playlists of music individualized to a person's tastes and preferences played directly to the individual using earphones or various other digital devices. This music is able to tap into deep-seated memories, enabling them to sing along with their favorite tunes, become more engaged with the environment, and more conversant with those around them: fellow residents, staff, and loved ones. Individuals exposed to the program are more calm and responsive to those around them, which has been reported to help in the reduced use of antipsychotic medications. As of 2016, The Music and Memory program was being utilized in three thousand of the over 15,000 nursing homes in the U.S. You can find more at https://musicandmemory.org.

The Music and Memory Program is based on the award- winning documentary *Alive Inside*, which was an Audience Choice Award winner at the 2014 Sundance Film Festival. The movie director, Michael Rossato Bennett, chronicled Dan Cohen's work over a period of three years and showed that music has the ability to help people not only connect with their memories but also with who they are. *Alive Inside* can be streamed online on Amazon Prime.

In addition to gaps in communication and the inability to recall specific words, speech may become more mumbled, and then quiet or even nonexistent as the disease progresses, making it even more difficult to understand. Individual personality characteristics may also play a role. If one was timid, soft-spoken, and reluctant to express themselves prior to onset of the disease, they may be even more likely to "act" that way as they experience more difficulty communicating. However, for the person who was outgoing, verbal, and assertive, it may represent a major change from their personality. This person may "elect" to talk less, seeming to them becoming resolved to letting things happen around them. Imagine this scenario:

> You are home alone or working alone in an office, when suddenly, out of the clear blue sky, you feel an itch in the middle of your back. You struggle over and over again to stretch your arms across your back to reach the spot. It becomes maddening, trying to reach that darn itch you cannot get rid of. You start looking for things that you could hold in your hand to reach it—a ruler, a spatula, anything long enough. You start feeling desperate. You go to the edge of a doorway and try rubbing your back to and fro against it to try and get rid of that darn itch. NOTHING IS WORKING! Finally, someone comes along and you ask them to scratch your back. You give them clear directions,

telling them to move their hand up, down, right, left, until finally, aah, they find the spot and scratch that darn itch until it is gone. You let out a loud sigh of relief, "Aaaahhhhhh!" The feeling is unbelievable.

Now consider the same scenario, but imagine that you are unable to tell anyone you have an itch. You cannot find the words or describe to them how to reach that area of your back so you can get some relief. How would you feel? What would you do? How would you act? Consider also that you are confused and in unfamiliar surroundings with people scurrying around you, not paying much attention to how you are feeling or what you need, or even whether or not you are even there.

Though research and writing about dementia has become increasingly visible in the literature since the early 2000s, a book entitled *Holding on to Home: Designing Environments for People with Dementia*[91] was written in 1991, which predated Dr. William Thomas' book on the Green House Project and his experiments at Chase Memorial Nursing Home. The authors work described designing an environment more appropriately suited to caring for individuals with Alzheimer's disease and dementia. In fact, they advocated for a setting that was more akin to a home environment in favor of the traditional institutional type nursing home environment with long hallways and wards or units which they described as a "junior hospital" They advocated for living spaces with a living room, dining room, kitchen, and activity room and optimally could include a restaurant, movie theatre, art studio, exercise room, and pool. While the latter amenities may seem like luxuries and not necessarily feasible, the importance of providing a more homelike environment is a realistic consideration. This, as far back as 1991. How many living spaces, nursing homes, etc have been designed or built since that time and how many of them have taken that valuable insight into consideration when designing a space for individuals with Alzheimer's disease or dementia?

Subsequent studies beginning from the early 2000s discussed the importance of the physical environment as a contributing factor to behaviors associated with increased confusion. A review of the literature found that, though a secure environment with specific boundaries and safety features was obviously important, negative responses were found in environments where security features obstructed the freedom of movement. In addition, individuals with dementia were reported to experience a higher quality of life in buildings in which they have access to both indoor and outdoor activities, provide opportunity for privacy as well as social engagement with others whether in the facility or the community, and have the opportunity to engage with familiar activities, especially those that are domestic in nature.

Despite the best intentions of family and loved ones who want to continue caring for the individual with Alzheimer's disease or dementia at home, there may be times when it becomes increasingly difficult and no longer possible. Families want their loved one to have the best care possible in the safest environment but realize that they can no longer provide that. There may be guilt associated with that decision but also an understanding of the difficulties involved in meeting their loved one's needs emotionally, psychologically, physically, and medically. They are, therefore, in the untenable position of placing their trust in those that are caring for their loved one in a facility.

I think it is a fair statement that many facilities are not yet equipped with the understanding or willingness to provide what is needed for individuals who suffer from either dementia or Alzheimer's disease. While there are efforts underway, especially in Massachusetts, this will take time to become part of the fabric of the typical nursing home environment. Many staff members who work in facilities are doing the best they can with the help and training that is available to them. The best course of action may be to present yourself as a care partner with the staff. The adage, "You catch more flies with honey than with vinegar," is certainly apt for this situation. After all, it is hard for families and friends to deal with the symptoms associated with the disease.

Most people that find themselves admitted to a facility, including those with Alzheimer's disease or dementia, experience a loss of control or independence. Therefore, it is most beneficial if staff approaches people in a way that helps them feel empowered in an effort to mitigate the sense of loss of independence and loss of control. This is often when people become even more angry or frustrated and tend to "act out." It makes perfect sense. They have no say in their care and daily routine.

Therefore, upon visiting any facility, one should observe how the staff talks to the residents. Are they "ordering them around" with directives such as: "It's time to eat," "It's time for you to get up," or "I'm taking you to the birthday party now." Are they pushing people in wheelchairs mindlessly without even informing them where they are taking them or what they are going to be doing. I've unfortunately witnessed this situation many times.

One thing is for sure, if an individual with dementia is approached in a way that is uncomfortable or unfamiliar, they may react in a way that is considered to be "acting out" behavior. Observing staff interactions with residents already living in the facility is one way to determine how your loved one will be treated in this facility.

Think of children who cannot express feeling tired, in pain, angry, hurt, etc. Parents and other adults interpret their behaviors, assigning what they think may remedy the situation. How many of us have seen a cranky, restless, crying child and have interpreted that behavior to mean that he or she may be feeling tired? How many teachers have seen a child acting out in a classroom and discerned that they may be feeling hungry, experiencing some type of family or personal situation, or having learning difficulties because of some undiagnosed deficit? Why do we not apply the same level of understanding to adults who are experiencing mental decline associated with Alzheimer's disease or dementia?

When your loved one enters the long-term care unit of a long-term care facility, you will encounter a variety of personnel that will be responsible for their direct medical, nursing, and clinical care. A primary care physician will be assigned to the unit where your loved one will be living who will oversee the care. This doctor should be a geriatrician, a doctor who is trained in working with people with Alzheimer's disease and related dementias and the conditions associated with aging. You should feel free to ask if that is the case.

Many people with dementia sometimes find themselves feeling depressed, angry, and scared. This could be compounded by being placed in a nursing home facility, separated from family and friends, away from familiar surroundings and facing the loss of independence. This also can exacerbate the confusion they are already experiencing. An important member of the team may be a psychiatrist and/or psychologist. They should be readily available to visit your loved one on the memory care unit. However, the all-important issue of prescribing antipsychotic drugs by these health professionals as the treatment of choice is one that loved ones must be aware of, and question, as the need arises.

There is typically a nurse who manages the dementia unit. This person should be a registered nurse (RN) who is experienced working with patients with Alzheimer's disease or dementia. Find out how long they have been working on the unit and how long they have been working at the facility. There also will be other nurses on the unit: a licensed practical nurse (who is usually assigned to dispensing the prescribed medications) and certified nursing assistants, the practitioners who will have the most contact with your loved one and provide most of the daily care. The training they receive and experience they have working with patients with Alzheimer's disease and dementia are also critically important.

The role of the speech pathologist can be an important one for the person with Alzheimer's disease or dementia. The facility should have a speech pathologist who is available to provide therapy as needed and appropriate for your loved one. The speech therapist will work with your loved one to maximize communication and cognitive functioning, educate the staff on the specific strategies your loved one requires, and will also be able to address changing eating or swallowing issues that often arise as the disease progresses. They may alter the consistency of the food for your loved one and also can educate the staff on appropriate techniques if assistance with feeding is required.

Occupational and physical therapists should also be available to address mobility and flexibility issues and activities of daily living (eating, bathing, toileting, and grooming). They will provide therapy to your loved one as needed, and they will also direct and educate the staff on the best ways to maintain optimal functioning while providing assistance in each of these areas.

It is important to visit any facility prior to placing your loved one who has dementia or Alzheimer's disease. The following is a suggested list of questions you should ask. Of course, you may have others.

- What specific activities do you provide for individuals with Alzheimer's disease or dementia?

- Do you have an activities specialist assigned to that unit?

- What is that person's training to work with Alzheimer's disease or dementia?

- How often do you have activities for this unit? What are the patients doing, or how are they engaged, outside of scheduled activities?

- What kinds of specific activities are in place to address the behaviors and confusion that are associated with dementia or Alzheimer's disease? Is there a continuum of activities provided to accommodate confusion as it progresses?

- Are residents encouraged to attend off-unit activities so they can interact with other residents of the facility?

- If they are unable to do so, or if they don't want to go, how is that handled? How are they engaged if they remain on the unit?

- Do you provide assistance with meals?

- Is there a secure outdoor space? Are residents taken out of doors on a regular basis?

- How many nurses and staff members are on the unit at any given time throughout the day, evening, nights, and weekends?

- What specialized training does the staff on the unit (RNs, LPNs, CNAs) receive in order to work with Alzheimers's/dementia patients? What about other staff members who interact with the residents on the unit (including porters and dietary aides)? What specialized training have they received? How often is the training offered?

- How is the resident oriented to the unit and to the other residents? To the person(s) with whom they share a room (if two-bedded or multi-bedded rooms)?

- Are the hallways wide enough to allow for residents to walk around?

- Are residents free to, and encouraged to, walk around as long as they are able?

- How do you handle residents who "forget" where their room is located or wander into other residents' rooms?

- How do you handle acting out behavior? What do you think are the root or underlying causes?

One of the most helpful resources in finding a long-term care facility that understands the needs of the person is Pioneer Network. As I noted in chapter seven, It is an organization that stands for placing the needs and preferences of the individual first and foremost in the care model. The facilities they recommend deviate from the norm of what exists in most facilities to date. They represent a change in culture, not only of the nursing home industry, but for how we care for the elder citizens in our society. When I discovered Pioneer Network I felt as though I found a chorus of voices beautifully singing the same song.

Alzheimer's Legislation

In August 2018, the governor of Massachusetts signed an act concerning Alzheimer's disease and associated dementias which had unanimously passed the Senate and House of Representatives earlier in the year. Statistics indicate that "more than 130,000 people are currently living with Alzheimer's disease in Massachusetts—those individuals are being cared for by more than 337,000 family and friends. According to the Alzheimer's Association, in 2018 Massachusetts will spend more than $1.6 billion in Medicaid costs caring for people with Alzheimer's."[92]

The legislation was signed on the back of allocating $100,000 to increase public awareness about the disease. In addition, Governor Baker, together with the governor of Montana, wrote an op-ed piece essentially encouraging the federal government to understand the need to allocate resources at the state level to address this disease that is growing by leaps and bounds in our population.

As Massachusetts has taken a leadership role in healthcare legislation over the years, the case with this legislation is no different. My hope is that it will set the trend for other states to take action to allocate the necessary resources to help both the patients and their families who are dealing with Alzheimer's disease. Certainly, it highlights the need for that to happen.

As stated by Daniel Zotos, director of Public Policy and Advocacy of the Massachusetts/New Hampshire Chapter of the Alzheimer's Association: "Alzheimer's is the single largest unaddressed public health threat in the 21st century."[93] It truly is a growing issue for US ALL.

Alzheimer's disease and dementia are a reality. If our loved ones experience either of these conditions, we must find constructive ways to help them through the associated issues, including the confusion and anger that may arise when one loses his or her memory. People with Alzheimer's disease and dementia require care and understanding. It is vital that when we entrust them to someone's care, those individuals are properly trained, competent professionals who are sensitive to the extra attention and patience needed. They must be able to render care with appropriate understanding, empathy, and compassion. We must always be vigilant in our choices of care for our elders. This is especially true when their vulnerability is related to Alzheimer's disease and dementia.

Federal Legislation

On December 31, 2018, the president signed a $100 million bill into law that was cosponsored by half of the members of the House of Representatives and the Senate. The legislation is known as Building Our Largest Dementia (BOLD) Infrastructure for Alzheimer's Act. The bill, which was first introduced in November 2017, authorizes government spending of $20 million/year for each of five years in the area of Alzheimer's education, research, treatment and improved care. This is a momumental and important step to address the burgeoning population afflicted with Alzheimer's disease which is projected by *Alzheimer's News Today* to skyrocket to as high as 16 million by 2050. This is estimated to represent annual spending of the federal budget to more than $1.1 trillion.

NINE

SYSTEMIC ADVOCACY VERSUS GRASSROOTS ADVOCACY

We all require and want respect,
man or woman, black or white.
It's our basic human right.
ARETHA FRANKLIN

The above quote applies to us all, but it particularly speaks to the issue of how we care for our elder citizens:

What Is Systemic Advocacy?

Systemic advocacy is a process that seeks to influence and change a "system." Examples of systems might be legislative or government policy and may even extend to community attitudes. Lobbying efforts are a form of systemic advocacy that presents attempts to exert influence for or against an issue to legislators or government officials.

What Is Grassroots Advocacy?

Grassroots advocacy is usually intended to reach the general public, asking them to take some kind of action. One form of action might be to contact their legislators and government officials to express their opinion about a particular issue to influence them to take legislative action. In this manner, grassroots advocacy exerts its influence to create systemic change. However, another way that grassroots advocacy can be effective is to create a public outcry loud enough that it will bring the topic to the forefront of the national conversation. This outcry can create a groundswell movement that will ultimately affect public awareness of the importance of the issue in order to bring about social change.

Grassroots advocacy has been an effective vehicle to bring about social and legislative changes throughout the history of our country. The civil rights movement is one example. One of the precipitative events that led to the beginning of desegregation in the United States was the arrest of Rosa Parks on December 1, 1955. As a result of her arrest, the Montgomery Bus Boycott of December 5, 1955, was born when 90 percent of the black citizens of Montgomery, Alabama, started to refuse to ride the buses. This thirteen-month-long mass protest culminated in the U.S. Supreme Court ruling that segregation on public buses is unconstitutional.

Other issues have taken root in our national conversation that began with the voices of outspoken individuals. These individual voices led to more voices, until the number of individual voices became a loud collective voice that could not be ignored. I'm thinking of issues such as AIDS, heart disease, women's rights (most notably the recent #MeToo movement), drug addiction (including the opioid crisis), mental illness, depression, and Alzheimer's disease.

The issue of long-term care and how we treat our elder citizens, specifically, has not yet been addressed.

To reiterate, there are over 15,000 nursing homes or skilled nursing facilities in the U.S. in which over 1.5 million of our elder citizens reside. These are our grandparents and parents, aunts, uncles, sisters, brothers, husbands and wives. While there are functioning alternative models of new and better ways to care for our elder citizens, these are the exception, not the norm.

What Is Being Done in Terms of Systemic Advocacy and Who Is Doing It?

There are national organization that are addressing important issues in order to effect change through legislative and government channels.

The National Consumer Voice for Quality Long Term Care, colloquially known as *The Consumer Voice*, is a nonprofit organization that promotes awareness of issues relating to long-term care. It analyzes government policy and plays an important role in systemic advocacy, promoting issues related to nursing home reform and quality care to legislators and government agencies. The information it provides is useful for consumers, families, caregivers, and advocates. It offers instructions on how citizens can communicate with lawmakers to express their concerns about important legislation relating to elder citizen care. Another important facet of the organization is its work with the National Ombudsmen Program, which was created as an oversight body to ensure quality care and consumer rights for all nursing home residents. The Consumer Voice holds a yearly national conference in Alexandria, Virginia. The organization's motto is: "Quality Now: Consumer Rights Are Human Rights." (Contact: http://theconsumervoice.org)

A second important organization is the *Long-Term Care Community Coalition*, known by the acronym LTCCC. A nonprofit advocacy organization, its mission it is to address important issues related to quality of care and quality of life for elder citizens and those who are disabled, living in nursing homes, and assisted living centers. The organization also conducts research into policy matters and publishes fact sheets, articles, and newsletters in an effort to provide information to caregivers and families. The Long-Term Care Community Coalition is closely aligned with The Consumer Voice, and through its work also provides important information to politicians and government officials. Its motto is "Advancing Quality, Dignity & Justice." (Contact: http://nursinghome411.org)

One of the most widely known and visible organizations that advocates for senior citizens is *AARP* (American Association of Retired Persons.) Most people associate AARP with providing information on resources and discounts for a variety of goods and services sold in the community. But AARP has a more powerful role in the area of systemic advocacy by imploring legislators to remember the issues important to seniors when they are introducing legislation or voting on policies that would impact them. AARP is not limited to nursing homes/long-term care or assisted living facilities. Similar to The Consumer Voice, AARP also provides information to their constituents about important legislation of concern to them or their loved ones and offers methods for contacting their political leaders to weigh in with their opinions. (Contact: http://aarp.org)

National Council on Aging is a government agency that works hand in hand with nonprofit organizations and businesses to provide information and locate resources and benefits that elder citizens can access to make their lives easier. It also functions as a systemic advocacy organization in representing elder citizen issues at the policy level. The organization issues "advocacy alerts" so that those interested can receive information on the latest policy decisions and, as with The Consumer Voice, AARP provides helpful information on ways to get involved and let his/her voice be heard. (Contact: http://ncoa.org)

The Administration on Aging is strictly a government organization whose sole purpose is to advocate for the concerns of elder citizens. Its primary role is to maintain the issues of importance to elder citizens in the forefront of government organizations. It also provides grant money to organizations that provide direct services to elder citizens. (Contact: http://acl.gov)

Last, but not least, the *Alzheimer's Association* was created to address the needs and concerns of the ever-growing population of those affected by Alzheimer's disease in this country. To date that is slightly over 5 million (35.6 million worldwide). The Alzheimer's

Association reports that by 2025 that number will increase to 7.1 million people aged sixty-five and older affected by Alzheimer's disease. By 2050 that number is projected to jump to 16 million in the United States and 115.4 million people across the globe. With the anticipated increase in the number of Americans afflicted with Alzheimer's disease, there will be an even greater need for appropriate care. While many family members are extending every effort to care for their loved ones at home, there are situations when the need requires long-term care/ skilled nursing facility placement.

The Association is a systemic advocacy organization that promotes research, advocates for policies, and advocates for better care for those afflicted with the disease as well as their families. AARP recently donated $60 million to research into finding a cure and developing treatment for Alzheimer's disease and dementia. Bill Gates also donated $50 million of his own money to develop treatment for the disease. (Contact: http://alz.org)

The Pioneer Network, as I have noted in previous chapters, is considered to be a leader for changing the culture of aging in the United States. Its mission is *helping care providers transition away from a medical, institutional model of elder care to one that is life affirming, satisfying, humane and meaningful.* In doing so, it advocates that individual voices are heard and respected. Their goal is to transform the culture in health care organizations so that the care administered is directed by the person who is receiving it. (Contact: https://www. pioneernetwork.net)

The Fundamental Question

While all these associations and organizations are doing extremely important work in the area of aging, *a fundamental question* remains: With all of the organizations focused on systemic advocacy for the issues of importance to elder citizens, including the care provided to them in nursing home/skilled nursing facilities, why are we *not* doing a better job for the elder citizens that reside in these facilities?

As we know, the wheels of justice turn slowly. And where big money is concerned, the wheels turn even slower. The major players involved in the corporatization of the nursing home industry have the dollars and, as we all know, often carry the weight and the lion's share of the voice.

The industry is more and more structured *for-profit*.

It's not that the for-profit model cannot be maintained. The question is *to what degree?*

Must the driving force be to provide the least in order to gain the most? Must the drive for profit be so great that it outweighs the desire or willingness to provide in some cases even a modicum of an adequate quality of life?

I strongly believe that, as a society, we should be calling for a better situation for our elder citizens as they advance through the years so they can live with dignity until their last day.

I, therefore, am calling for *grassroots advocacy.*

> *Change will not come if we wait for some other person, or if we wait*
> *for some other time. We are the ones we've been waiting for.*
> *We are the change that we seek.*
> BARACK OBAMA

"Dignity and respect are the root cause of every serious labor struggle," stated Jane McAlevey in her article on the West Virginia teacher's strike.[94] That may be true, but it is also true that the fight for dignity and respect have been at the root of every major social struggle, going as far back as the origins of the United States. The Boston Tea Party, precursor to the Revolutionary War, was a political protest essentially fighting for dignity and respect when the settlers were taxed without representation. The fight for women's rights, minority rights, and every other oppressed group has been a fight for dignity and respect. What was the basis of the Nursing Home Reform Act? A cry for improved quality of care, *dignity*, and *respect* for nursing home residents. What remains lacking in our care of elder citizens? *Dignity and Respect.*

For example, how did the teachers of West Virginia in early 2018 get all of their demands met when the odds were stacked against them?

It began with the teachers of one district deciding to strike. They were told it was illegal. They could lose their jobs, have their wages docked, be jailed. They were undeterred. What followed was remarkable. Before long, the teachers from all fifty-five districts across West Virginia walked out on strike. Every public school in every district was forced to close. When it appeared as though the union compromised with the governor for acquiescing to only a portion of the demands, the teachers were not satisfied. They continued with their mission, chose to defy union leadership, and voted to continue to strike until the deal was voted on by both houses of the State Senate and the governor signed it into law. They stood in solidarity and marched by the thousands in solidarity all the way to the State Capitol. Upon victory, they chanted, "Who made history? We made history."

The strike by the teachers of West Virginia inspired teachers in other states to take action. Teachers in Oklahoma, Arizona, and Kentucky followed suit in solidarity and protests over wages and benefits.

This is reminiscent of the situation I referenced in Selma, Alabama, when the entire black population decided not to ride public transportation. The Montgomery Bus Boycott brought the system to its knees. Facing disaster from the loss of revenue, political leaders had to capitulate and integrate the public transportation system.

Why are these references important? Because they highlight the importance of strength *in numbers* and what can be accomplished when sheer numbers of voices band together in unison to demand what is right.

I contend that the lack of quality care, dignity, and respect of our elder citizens in general, and within skilled nursing facilities in particular, has reached crisis proportions.

The time for us to demand what is right is NOW!

Needed is advocacy that will literally take root if many, many voices insist that what we are doing and how we are doing it is not good enough for those that have contributed to our society for their entire lives and have given birth to a new generation of citizens . . . most of whom, hopefully, will themselves become elder citizens.

As an example of public advocacy, the following was recently posted on the LTCCC (Long Term Care Coordinating Council of San Francisco) website:[95]

What Nursing Home Residents Are Entitled to But Rarely Get
- A regulatory agency that preserves and expands resident rights, rather than rolling them back.
- A regulatory agency that works for residents, instead of calling the nursing home industry its "customers."
- A regulatory agency that prevents resident harm, rather than reacting to it after the harm occurs.
- An enforcement system that properly penalizes nursing homes when residents are harmed and when the minimum standards of care are violated.
- Nursing homes which follow the minimum standards of care.
- Nursing homes that have adequate staffing and low antipsychotic drug use.
- Nursing homes that provide life with dignity.
- Peace of mind.

A Call to Action

What can each one of us do to begin a campaign for grassroots advocacy? In each of the forty-plus rehabilitation centers or skilled nursing facilities in which I've worked, I encountered patients, residents, or family members who had legitimate complaints about the quality of care, the staffing, food, environment, or overall treatment they received. In addition, many who work in these facilities complain about the ownership's lack of caring for them or the residents, the lack of supplies, and lack of adequate staff which too often results in frustration, injuries, and burnout.

Most of these negative issues can be traced to the idea that the facility was part of a corporate-type ownership structure.

In addition, since the writing of my last book, *Nursing Homes to Rehabilitation Centers . . . What Every Person Needs to Know*, I have had the opportunity to speak with many people who have had loved ones in facilities, both within my local vicinity as well as around the country.

The story is always the same. Recently I had an encounter with a gentleman at a party. There were several people at the table, and we went around introducing ourselves to each other and talking about our respective professions. When I said I was a speech/language pathologist who worked in rehabilitation centers and skilled nursing facilities, one of the men began talking about a facility his mother entered after she broke her hip. According to his description, she was an alert, verbal, and feisty woman. He had found the facility on the Nursing Home Compare website and placed his mother there because of the five-star rating—nothing less for his mother! With the very next sentence, he began talking about the inadequate staffing and substandard care that his mother experienced within a few days of her arrival. After he began to describe the situation, I interrupted and said, "Here, let *me* tell you what happened there."

After I described what I knew his mother had encountered, he said to me, "You just said exactly what happened. You should write a book about it." I laughed and told him I already had. What stood out was that here we were in the Northeast, and the situation his mother encountered took place in a facility in Florida, where sadly things were no different.

As he recounted the remainder of the story, it struck me that his mother's approach to receiving what seemed to be improved care for the remainder of her stay was actually just what was needed nationwide. It turns out his mother was an outspoken woman, full of spirit. After a week of waiting almost an hour on several occasions to have her bell answered so she could use the bathroom, being served cold and unappetizing food, and having only one shower *since she arrived*, she propelled her wheelchair to the nursing station. She emphatically told the nurse, who staring at a computer screen and barely glanced up as she was addressed, that unless they were going to provide better care, an improved response to her immediate needs, and somehow serve her better food, she was going to call the Department of Health and the local newspaper! In addition, she told the nurse that as soon as her son came to visit her over the weekend, she would be leaving to go home. He told me his mother related that story to him almost word-for-word, and knowing her personality, he had no doubt that the situation took place just as she described. Of course, after that "tirade," for the duration of her forty-five-day stay, the situation improved drastically.

Each person residing in a skilled nursing facility, short-term rehabilitation center or nursing home who experiences a situation that represents poor or substandard care or what is considered a violation of what is right, or just, in terms of care, decency, respect, or environment, should, of course, first take their issue to the appropriate staff members of the administration of the facility (e.g, the nurse manager on the appropriate unit, the social worker, the director of nursing, the administrator). In the event the issue is not satisfactorily resolved, the facility's ombudsman would be the next appropriate party to contact. Ombudsman information for the facility, including the phone number, should be posted and clearly visible. In the event these steps do not resolve the issue, or at any stage of the process, the individual resident or family member is free to place a call to the Department of Health of the state in which the facility is located. I advocate that in the most egregious situations, consideration should be considered to other more public forms of outreach: Call in to local radio stations, newspapers, TV stations, or your local congressional representatives.

For those who wish to or are able: *Write articles!*

Make your voice heard.

Consider asking TV stations to do live reports outside of a facility where an egregious situation has taken place. Family and friends of loved ones in any facility where such a situation exists should do the same.

The greater the number of voices that are heard surrounding the issues our elder citizens face within these facilities, the louder those voices become, and the more they cannot be ignored.

Those grassroots voices from outside, together with those individuals and organizations working diligently and relentlessly on systemic advocacy on the inside, will hopefully effect change sooner than rather than later, ensuring a better and happier quality of life for us all!

Let's do this.

EPILOGUE

After completing the manuscript for this book, I began reading a book entitled *Life Worth Living* by William H. Thomas, MD. The book is about The Eden Alternative in Action.

I was astounded when I read the first line of the first paragraph of the introduction: "This book is an attack on conventional nursing home practice." Of course, I read on. The paragraph concludes with the following statement: "My concern is with the flawed definition of caring that underlies contemporary nursing home care and management." The author says that "nursing home residents and their families can use [the book] in the struggle to promote change."[96]

I immediately called and texted people I knew. This book was already written, I told them. I immediately felt a tinge of disappointment. Was my time, effort, hard work, and energy for naught? A friend colleague of mine who no longer works in skilled nursing facilities said, "Wait a minute. How come we've never heard about this book and we've been working in this industry for years? When was the book written?"

We were both flabbergasted when I checked the copyright date—1996.

"If you are seeing and saying the same things from all the facilities you've worked in," she said, "nothing much has changed. And you *should* be writing this book." The more I thought about what she said, it seemed to make perfect sense. After I hung up the phone, I felt a lot better on one hand, but appalled on the other. Here was a credible, intelligent doctor addressing these issues in 1996, but over twenty years later, the majority of the over 15,000 nursing homes across the country strikingly resemble what he describes. There have been legislative attempts to address some of the issues faced by individuals who live in nursing homes, but they are not necessarily applied in a way that offers the quality of life, quality of care, and dignity and respect that we want for our loved ones.

So much of what Dr. Thomas was saying in 1996 unfortunately still applies to today. He talks about residents being on therapy overload. There is an obsession with therapy, "bloated with therapy," as he puts it. And that was before Resource Utilization Group categories and Case Mix Index. But he also mentions the fact that measured, defined, and quantifiable treatments, along with specific services and prescription drugs is what really matters to facilities—because that's what brings in the revenue.

Dr. Thomas wrote that the "devotion to treatment is both misguided and deeply entrenched in the nursing home system. The problem lies in the ways nursing homes are organized."

He brings up the overuse of prescription drugs and antipsychotic medications, especially to address "behavioral" issues. That practice is still rampant today. He highlights the three plagues of nursing home existence: boredom, loneliness, and helplessness. That remains the hallmark of nursing home life. He calls for a genuine commitment to change course in order to address and provide an improved quality of life. Yet there has been no significant change in this across the industry as a whole.

He addresses compassion or caring by using the phrase that residents are "starving for care." While there are certainly a number of caring staff members who work in facilities, compassion and empathy overall remain in short supply.

He also addresses staff turnover. The systemic cycle that promotes poor care and lack of respect or commitment for the *employee*, stems from lack of respect, interest, commitment to the *residents*.

He likens nursing homes to other institutional settings: prisons and mental hospitals, where the days are segmented and routinized. Residents are told what to do, what it is time for, and where to go. Residents now have greater choice in whether or not they will participate in a particular activity, when or what they eat, and when they wake up or go to bed. However, these "choices" are still juxtaposed against the context of a highly routinized and programmed institutional atmosphere.

Activity choices are limited, predictable, and boring, and they serve more to meet regulatory requirements as opposed to meeting the need of the residents. Activity choices may have increased in variety from bowling, horse racing, and bingo, but they remain few and far between and don't address the wide range of interests of the population. There also are large gaps in the day when there is no "programming" and residents and patients are left idle, not by choice.

I have suggested a wide range of activities in many facilities, including gardening, a cooking club, woodworking, Jeopardy nights, a book club, and Scrabble or other board games. Not one of these were introduced in any of the facilities. Over the years, I have suggested an innovative 'wheelchair dancing' program, as I have a friend who started such a program. as well as a dancing or movement program for people with Alzheimer's Disease and dementia. Despite repeated suggestions and information on how these programs could be helpful to improving the quality of residents' lives, none of the above ideas for programs were ever acted upon in any facility in which I worked.

Dr. Thomas wrote that residents are not treated as being live human beings. He calls nursing home facilities "mausoleums for the living." I have called them the "land of the living dead" or warehouses where people are essentially waiting to die.

Dr. Thomas mentions that the situation is "compounded by social trends that are weakening the sense of obligation across generations." I addressed this in chapter two, "Elder Care: A Moral Dilemma." This situation has only exacerbated with the passing years. However, there may be progress in this area on the horizon. Advances in technology in the way of conference calls, Skype, and so on may reduce the need for the family to relocate for job opportunities. Families may be able to make the decision to remain closer to their aging parents.

Dr. Thomas mentions the pleasing names of facilities along with slick marketing brochures, expensive marketing programs, and honey-tongued narrators that woo unsuspecting "customers," giving them an impression of facilities that are more appealing when, in actuality, they continue to resemble sterile institutions akin to prisons, reform schools, military boot camps, and cloistered convents with their routinized and programmed daily lives. My experience is that this has only gotten worse over the years as major corporations compete with one another in order to fill beds and woo the highest paying Medicare customers. Towards that end they redesign lobbies, rehabilitation departments and rooms on short-term rehabilitation units towith high end furnishings and amenities. This is also known as "the chandelier effect."

Finally, in the closing sentence of the introduction, Dr. Thomas states: "Professionals can use [this book] to transform their facilities into human habitats." While there are facilities that have successfully transformed by adopting a philosophy more akin to the "Eden Alternative," this is no easy task, especially in the present climate of corporate nursing home ownership and the drive for maximizing profit.

This brings us back to the initial question: How will change occur? What will be the incentive? Who will make that happen? The answer comes back to the initial answer: it is up to US! Each one of us need to insist on something better for ourselves, for our loved ones, and for our elder citizens.

APPENDIX

QUESTIONS TO ASK

When visiting a facility for a short-term rehabilitation placement, make sure you tour the long-term units even if you think your loved one is going to return home. This may take some convincing. Many admission directors will try to fiercely discourage you from visiting those areas. You may have to insist. I have known professionals going for a job interview who had to insist to see an entire building, even though the patients they were going to treat were on the short-term rehabilitation unit. The reasons are twofold:

Firstly, there are unanticipated situations that emerge that you cannot foresee which may cause circumstances to change. In that case, a short-term may lead to a long-term care stay.

This leads us to the second reason which is actually the most important. As you tour the building, you can observe and compare the surroundings of the short-term rehabilitation and long-term care units. How different are these areas in appearance?

It will give you a glimpse into the owners' perspective and how they view long-term residents as opposed to short-term patients. Is it all just for show just to get you in the door for the short-term Medicare dollars?

The following is a list of questions to consider asking when you visit any of these buildings. Don't forget: the facility is a business, you are visiting, and they now have, or will have, empty beds that they *must* fill. You are the buyer and they want your business. Some of the questions are repeated from the chapter on Alzheimer's Disease/Dementia because they are areas of concern applicable when touring a facility on any unit (short-term, long-term, or memory care unit).

- What is the staffing on the short-term rehabilitation unit? What is the staffing on the long-term care unit? *This should include information regarding RNs, LPNs and CNAs. Remember the law requires that an RN be on duty at least eight hours a day, seven days a week. Furthermore, facilities that have been identified as having reduced weekend staffing are not in compliance with regulations and as such can be cited for noncompliance.*

  - What is the daytime staffing on each of the units?"

  - What is the evening staffing?"

  - What is the weekend staffing?"

  - How many Registered Nurses (RN) are in the entire building per shift? What role do they play? *For example, in the evening, is the evening supervisor the only RN and is that person responsible for the entire building?*

- What is the staff turnover rate? *This will give you a glimpse into how satisfied the staff is with the administration and ownership. It usually has a direct relationship. The happier and more satisfied the staff, the more likely they will remain in a building for a longer period of time. This will tell you if your loved one can expect to have a consistent caregiver.*

- How often is a medical doctor in the facility?

- Does the building have mostly Physician Assistants or Nurse Practitioners caring for the patients? How often are they in the building?

- How many patients are the average caseload for the social workers in the building? Are they Clinical Social Workers? If they are clinical social workers, are they available to provide counselling and or supportive services?

- Do they have psychology or psychiatry services available the building? How often?

- What activities do they have for residents to address boredom and loneliness? How often are activities scheduled? *Ask for a list of the current week's activities and a calendar of the month's activities as well as a description of the activities offered.*

- Are there outside activities or excursions scheduled? How often? *Ask for examples.*

- What alternative activities does the building have suited to a patient's individual interests or level of cognition?

- Are there any specialty therapies available in the building? (e.g., pet therapy, aromatherapy) How often? *Ask for a description of what they entail. A pet coming to a facility once a week for a few minutes does not provide effective pet therapy.*

- How do they interpret, and respond to, behaviors of confused residents specifically, but residents in general? *Example: do they view the behavior as a person's attempt to communicate pain, discomfort, hunger, loneliness, boredom, etc.*

- How do they manage patients who become increasingly confused? What is the policy and procedure for prescribing antipsychotic drugs? What percentage of residents in the building are taking antipsychotic medications?

- Do they have a dementia or memory care unit? What does it consist of?

- What kinds of specific activities are in place to address the behaviors and confusion that are associated with dementia or Alzheimer's disease? Is there a continuum of activities provided to accommodate confusion as it progresses?

- What specialty services come to the building? Dental, vision, podiatry—how often are those specialists scheduled to come to the building?

- Where do they refer patients for other specialty services? (e.g., Neurology, Cardiac, Orthopedic)

- How many falls have occurred in the facility in the past six months?

Recent Medicare Changes

Positive

The Centers for Medicare and Medicaid Services has updated the policy for families and Medicare beneficiaries who have been denied continuation of therapy services based on lack of improvement. They have updated the policy to provide individuals and families with information on responding to, and appealing those denials. The denials were based on erroneous information that the individual can only continue to receive therapy services if they continue to make improvement. The regulations actually state that one does not need to improve in order continue receiving services. This was established in a case known as the *Jimmo v Sebelius Settlement*.

The settlement stipulates that those with specific medical conditions may receive ongoing skilled therapy in order to maintain their current level of function. Individuals that qualify for these services are those who have the following conditions: multiple dclerosis, Alzheimer's disease, Parkinson's disease, ALS (Lou Gehrig's disease), diabetes, hypertension, arthritis, heart disease, and stroke. There may be other serious conditions that would also qualify under this settlement. It is important to be aware of this information in the event an individual with one or any of the above conditions is discontinued from therapy due to lack of progress.

The New Jimmo Resources for the Center for Medicare Advocacy and the John A. Hartford Foundation can be viewed at http://www. medicareadvocacy.org/new-resources-from-the-center-for-medicare-advocacy-and-the-john-a-hartford-foundation.

Skilled Nursing Facility Expedited Appeals Checklist

This checklist provides an overview of the expedited appeals process that focuses on the termination of skilled care solely based on this erroneous "Improvement Standard." This can help Medicare beneficiaries and their families in their appeal process when receiving improper and unfair terminations and denials. It also outlines the criteria for coverage at a skilled nursing facility. The checklist can be viewed at: http://www.medicareadvocacy.org/wp-content/uploads/2018/09/Expedited-Appeals-Fact-Sheet.pdf

Skilled Nursing Facility Coverage Checklist

The settlement also stipulated that the Centers for Medicare & Medicaid Services revise the Medicare Benefit Policy Manual to clearly and unequivocally state that residents of a skilled nursing facility need not continue to improve in order for their care to be covered by Medicare. This information may be viewed at: http://www.medicareadvocacy.org/wp-content/uploads/2018/08/Checklist.pdf

Of importance to note: I emailed this information to several colleagues who are directors of rehabilitation departments in skilled nursing/rehabilitation center facilities, as well as to a friend who is part owner of a company that owns a small number of nursing homes. Each of these professionals denied knowing this information. This is why it is crucial for individual patients/residents and their families to be aware of the regulations and their rights under the law.

The Stamp Out Elder Abuse Act of 2018

Introduced by both Senate and House legislators thereby creating a semi-postal stamp to help as an additional funding source for federal government programs that address elder abuse, neglect and exploitation. These programs will include prevention, education, data collection, victim support and protection services and demonstration projects at both the Administration on Aging and Department of Justice. There will also be a path to investigate with the potential of prosecutorial action to anyone who perpetrates elder abuse or exploitation. "The menace of elder abuse continues in America" according to the press release by the Elder Justice Coalition, that National Advocacy Voice for Elder Justice in America. The press release states that according to the Department of Justice, one in ten elders in our country experiences elder abuse.

Residents Rights Month

Residents Rights Month occurs in October. Governors and mayors from municipalities in the following states: Florida, Georgia, Washington, D.C., Colorado, and Arizona have moved to officially proclaim October as Residents Rights Month. This is essential to underscore the guaranteed rights to all residents as it relates to dignity, choice, and self-determination as stipulated in the Nursing Home Reform Law of 1987. Find out if your state or local official has proclaimed October as Resident's Rights Month and press them to do so if they haven't already. I reached out to several rehabilitation directors, administrators, and personnel at the organizational level of the facilities with which I am acquainted. Each one of them seemed totally unaware of its existence.

Negative

In my previous book, *Nursing Homes to Rehabilitation Centers: What Every Person Needs to Know*, I referenced the tragedy at Hollywood Hills Nursing Home in Florida following Hurricane Irma in September

2017. Multiple people died, essentially suffocating, because of the lack of electricity and ventilation at the facility.

While the report of the tragedy and Hollywood Hills became part of a passing news cycle, thankfully, it was recognized as an extremely serious matter by politicians and advocacy organizations. In response to pressure from these groups, the Centers for Medicare and Medicaid Services took action and instituted revised emergency preparedness regulations for all providers and suppliers that participate in receiving Medicare and Medicaid reimbursement. The finalized rule was published on September 16, 2016, as 81 FR 63860. The regulations became effective in November 2016; the full Emergency Preparedness Regulations were issued in June 2017 as Appendix Z of the Standard Operations Manual. They were to be implemented by November 2017. The fact that there was such a swift response to this tragedy was gratifying.

Fast-forward to Monday, September 17, 2018, when I received a press release via email from the Centers for Medicare and Medicaid Services with the following headline: "CMS Proposes to Lift Unnecessary Regulations and Ease Burden on Providers."

This headline was particularly unsettling because in my mind it raised the all-to familiar issue of CMS' provider concerns. Of course, it was veiled in the context of lifting and easing unnecessary regulations which would ultimately result in improved quality care. I was admittedly suspicious before even reading it. When I read through the ruling, my suspicions were confirmed in at least one area: "CMS is proposing rolling back Emergency Preparedness Rules."

I could not believe my eyes. Only ten months after the implementation of the Emergency Preparedness Rules, the Centers for Medicare and Medicaid Services issued a proposed ruling revising these regulations. According to the proposed ruling, this is part of an effort to "relieve burden on healthcare providers by removing unnecessary, obsolete or excessively burdensome Medicare compliance requirements for healthcare facilities." The information was contained in a document entitled. "Medicare and Medicaid Programs; Regulatory Provisions to Promote Program Efficiency, Transparency, and Burden Reduction"[97]

A review of the press release finds that the Centers for Medicare and Medicaid services proposes to revise the requirements so that providers have "increased flexibility with compliance." Most of the changes involve reducing the time frames in which facilities must review and update their emergency preparedness plans, policies, and procedures, training, and testing from one year to every two years. For instance, the facility would only have to review and update its emergency preparedness plan, policies, and procedures, communication plan, and training and testing program at least every two years instead of annually. Furthermore, the original regulations state that each in-patient provider is required to conduct two annual testing exercises. The proposed rule expands the type of testing exercises a provider can choose to conduct for one of these annual exercises. The choices are as follows: "full-scale community-based exercise, if available; an individual facility-based functional exercise; a drill, or a tabletop exercise; or workshop that includes a group discussion led by a facilitator."[98]

From my experience, I don't think it's entirely unfair to assume that many facilities would choose the least costly and least intrusive into the day-to-day workings of the facility: a tabletop exercise or a group-discussion workshop. A proposed change in the regulation also states that after initially training staff, a facility would only be required to conduct training every two years, rather than the present annual requirement. The impracticality and harmful effects this represents to patients and residents in facilities cannot be overstated. Staff turnover is an issue that is acknowledged as a problem in most facilities; how then will the staff be prepared if they are not trained on a regular basis? CMS also proposes to eliminate part of the requirement for both hospitals and Medicare and Medicaid provider facilities regarding their collaboration and cooperation with local emergency preparedness agencies and officials in the event of a disaster or emergency. They will continue to be required to participate and work with those officials, but they will no longer be required to provide documentation that they have done so. Therefore, if documentation does not have to be provided, it is up to the conscience, caring, and good will of the administration of any particular facility to adhere to their responsibility in this area. I am extremely suspect of the elimination of the requirement in this area. Can we trust the administration and ownership to participate in these functions? Is this any different than relying on facility administration to accurately report their staffing in order to get a high star rating on the Nursing Home Compare website? Have we not depended on administration good will to do the right thing long enough?

It is disheartening to think that, once again, the Centers for Medicare and Medicaid Services responded to the "burden and expense" it represents to providers as superseding the value of human life. I can't imagine how any reasonably thinking person can consider anything less than an annual emergency preparedness policy review and training to not be harmful.

As I was writing this, North and South Carolina were experiencing the devastating effects of Hurricane Florence. In the aftermath of Hurricane Irma in Florida, is this the time to "water-down" implementation of regulations that were designed to save people's lives? Does the reasoning to reduce the cost and expense, which providers consider to be a burden, make any sense when juxtaposed against people's lives? Is this what we want for our parents?

Respond to the Federal government in any way you can. Contact your local Congressional representative and/or senator. Place phone calls to government agencies. Tell them this is unacceptable!

Be an advocate for your loved ones and our elderly population. It's time to speak out loudly and demand the change the must occur as a larger percentage of our population ages. We all deserve dignity and respect. It is our right—no matter how old or infirm we are.

NOTES

1. Health Care Financing Administration, Office of the Actuary, Data from the Office of National Health Statistics in Health Care Financing Review, Fall 1994, Vol. 16, No. 1. & Commission on Long-Term Care (2013). Report to Congress, Washington, D.C. Sept. 30.

2. Hawes C. and Phillips, C.D. "The Changing Structure of the Nursing Home Industry and the Impact of Ownership on Quality, Cost, and Access," last modified 1986, accessed May 2017, https://www.ncbi.nlm.nih.gov/books/NBK217907/.

3. "Poorly Performing Nursing Homes: Special Focus Facilities are Often Improving, but CMS's Program Could Be Strengthened," US Government Accountability Office, last modified April 19, 2010, accessed May 2017, http://www.gao.gov/products/ GAO -10 -197.

4. "Nursing Homes Private Investment Homes Sometimes Differ from Others in Deficiencies, Staffing, and Financial Performance," US Government Accountability Office, last modified July 2011, accessed May 2017, http://www.gao.gov/new.items/ d11571.pdfancial.

5. https://www.ncmust.com/doclib/OBRA87summary.pdf.

6. Ibid.

7. Martin Luther King, Chicago Press Conference, March 25, 1966, in connection with the annual meeting of Medical Committee of Human Rights.

8. https://en.newsner.com/family/woman-dies-in-nusing-home-then-nurse-finds-a-note-that-brings-everyone-to- tears-will-nurse-a-note-concerning-all-the-tears/.

9. Mahoney, M., "Ageism in Health Care Estimated to Cost $63 Billion Annually" Yale News, Nov 14, 2018.

10. Wikipedia, s.v. "Old Age," accessed October 2016, https://en.wikipedia.org/wiki/ Old age.

11. Older People Projected to Outnumber Children - Census

Bureauhttps://www.census.gov/newsroom/press.../cb18-41-population-projections.html and The Graying of America: More Older Adults Than ... - Census Bureauhttps://www.census.gov/library/stories/2018/03/graying-america.html.

12. World Population Ageing - UN.orgwww.un.org/en/development/desa/population/publications/.../WPA2015_Report.pdf.

13. O. Wright, "'Our National Shame': Health Secretary Jeremy Hunt Blasts British Society's Neglect of Its Elderly," Independent, last modified October 17, 2013, accessed October 2016, http://www.independent.co.uk/news/uk/politics/our-national-shame-health-secretary-jeremy-hunt-blasts-british-society-s-neglect-of-its-elderly-8887532.html.

14. D. Blackburn, "Jeremy Hunt Calls for 'Profound Transformation in the Culture' of the NHS," *The Spectator*, November 19, 2013, accessed January 2017, https://blogs. spectator.co.uk/.

15. "Filial Piety Sutra, The Sutra about the Deep Kindness of Parents and the Difficulty of Repaying It," abstracted from the translation by Upasika Terri Nicholson, as reviewed by Bhikshuni Heng Tao, edited by Bhikshuni Heng Ch'ih and Upasika Susuan Rounds, and certified by Abbot Hua and Bhikshuni Heng Tao. *YBAM Buddhist Digest*, accessed October 2016, http://oaks.nvg.org/filial-piety.html.

16. M. Meng M. and Hunt, K. "New Chinese Law: Visit Your Parents," CNN, last modified July 2, 2013, accessed November 2016, www.cnn.com/2013/07/02/world/asia/china- elderly-law/index.html.

17. Chan, quoting Confucius in Analects, W., *Source Book in Chinese Philosophy* (Princeton, NJ: Princeton University Press, 1963).

18. "Seven Cultures that Celebrate Aging and Respect Their Elders," *Huffington Post*, last modified May 16, 2015, accessed November 2016, https://www.huffington-post.com/2014/02/25/what-other-cultures-can-teach_n_4834228.html.

19. White Feather, "Native American Beliefs," *Inter-Tribal Times*, last modified October 1994, accessed December 2016, http://www. home.earthlink.net/~tessia/Native.html, (hereafter cited as "Native American Beliefs").

20. C. Printup-Harms, C. "Aging Elders Among Native American Populations," Niagara County New York, accessed December 2016, http://www.niagaracounty.com/Portals/5/ Images/June2010.pdf.

21. "Native American Beliefs."

22. Ward, B. "Third Generation Country, A Practical Guide to Raising Children with Great Values," accessed January 2017, https:// www.values.com/inspirational- quotes/3002-we-were-taught-to-respect-elders-.

23. D. Lelvada, "How Two Organizations Are Bringing Hope and Care to Greece's Elderly," *Huffington Post*, last modified January 10, 2017, accessed May 2017, www. huffingtonpost.com/entry/greece-elderly_us_561d6ed5e4b0c5a1ce60f1d2.

24. Wilsher, K. "French Forced to Care for Elderly Parents," Fairfax Digital, last modified February 16, 2004, accessed October 2016, http://www.theage.com.au/ articles/2004/02/15/1076779835689. html (hereafter cited as "French Forced to Care for Elderly Parents").

25. "French Forced to Care for Elderly Parents."

26. "French Forced to Care for Elderly Parents."

27. "Open-Ended Working Group on Ageing," United Nations Human Rights Office of the High Commissioner, accessed April 2017, https://social.un.org/ ageing-working-group/.

28. Krantz, M. "Wall Street Banks Ace Fed's Severe Stress Test," *USA Today* Money Section B, June 24, 2016, p.1.

29. McKoy, K. "Bank of America fined $430M for Cash Misuse," *USA Today* Money Section B, June 24, 2016, p.2.

30. Mongan, E. "Illinois Becomes the Fifth State to Allow Cameras in Nursing Home Rooms," McKnights: The News You

Need, accessed August 2015, http://www.mcknights. com/news/illinois-becomes-fifth-state-to-allow-cameras-in-nursing-home-rooms/article/434524/?webSyncID=2a2109e8-d644-2377-448a-0398bb1508d7&sessionGUID=2c8 a31c4-ad18-09e7-58c5-12b202da724d.

31. "Nursing Home Residents at Risk," The Long-Term Care Community Coalition, accessed June 2017, http://www.ltccc.org.

32. Pear, R. "Violations Reported at 94% of Nursing Homes," *New York Times*, September 29, 2008 accessed February 2017, www.nytimes.com/2008/09/30/us/30nursing.html.

33. Ochinko, W. "Nursing Home Quality: Findings from GAO Reports," National Health Policy Forum, accessed August 2017, http://www.nhpf.org/library/handouts/ Ochinko.slides_03-25-10.pdf.

34. Abramo, A. and Lehman, J. "How N.Y.'s Biggest For-Profit Nursing Home Group Flourishes Despite a Record of Patient Harm," ProPublica, last modified October 27, 2015, accessed October 2016, https://www.propublica.org/article/new-york-for-profit-nursing-home-group-flourishes-despite-patient-harm (hereafter cited as "How N.Y.'s Biggest For-Profit Nursing Home Group Flourishes Despite a Record of Patient Harm").

35. R. "Sentosa Care's Expansion in NY," Abuse and Neglect, Advocacy, Staffing and Trial Themes, accessed October 2016, http://www.gpoliakoff.com/.

36. "How N.Y.'s Biggest For-Profit Nursing Home Group Flourishes Despite a Record of Patient Harm."

37. "How N.Y.'s Biggest For-Profit Nursing Home Group Flourishes Despite a Record of Patient Harm."

38. Mollot, R. "Executive Summary: Safeguarding Residents and Program Integrity in NY State Nursing Homes," The Long-Term Care Community Coalition, last modified 2015, accessed September 2017, http://nursinghome411.org/?s=safeguarding.

39. If you are interested in finding more specific information on the New Long-Term Care survey, visit the following link under the heading Downloads: New Long-Term Care Survey Process-Slide Deck and Speaker Notes; https://www.cms.gov/Medicare/Provider-Enrollment-and-Certification/GuidanceforLawsAndRegulations/Nursing- Homes.html.

40. Letter to CMS, October 31, 2017 The National Consumer Voice for Quality Long-Term Care, accessed November 2017, http://theconsumervoice.org/uploads/files/issues/CMS_letter_about_rollback_of_nursing_home_regulations_10-26-17.pdf.

41. Rau, J., "Feds Order More Weekend Inspections of Nursing Homes to Catch Understaffing," *Kaiser Health News*; https://khn.org/news/feds-order-more-weekend-inspections-of-nursing-homes-to-catch-understaffing/Nov 30, 2018.

42. Ostrov, B.F., "More than Half of California Nursing Homes Balk at Stricter Staffing Rules," *Kaisier Health News*; https://khn.org/news/more-than-half-of-california-nursing-homes-balk-at-stricter-staffing-rules/ Dec 7. 2018

43. "More than Half of California Nursing Homes Balk at Stricter Staffing Rules."

44. To learn more about the deficiency categories, you can visit: www.cms.gov/Medicare/Provider-Enrollment-and…/Nursing-Homes.html or www.cms.gov/Medicare/Provider-Enrollment/and…QSO18-18-NH.pdf.

45. St. Hilaire, A. "Report Finds that Lack of Enforcement Allowed for Neglect at State Nursing Homes," *ABC News*, Updated September, 2016, accessed November, 2016 http://abc27.com/2016/07/26/report-finds-that-lack-of-enforcement-allowed-for-neglect-at-state-nursing-homes.

46. Geri-chair is short for geriatric chair. It is a chair that reclines primarily used in medical facilities for patients after they recover from illness or surgery as well as for older more infirm individuals

who have difficulty sitting upright. It is a rather large padded chair that is more comfortable than a traditional chair. The chair rolls on large casters and can be adjusted from upright to the reclining position. Because of its size it is sometimes awkward to maneuver.

47. "Staffing Data Submission PBJ" Centers for Medicare & Medicaid Services Last modified 9/28/2017 accessed October 2017, https://www.cms.gov/Medicare/Quality-Initiatives-Patient-Assessment-Instruments/NursingHomeQualityInits/Staffing-Data-Submission-PBJ.html.

48. https://www.cms.gov/Medicare/Provider-Enrollment-and-Certification/CertificationandCompliance/downloads/users-guide.pdf.

49. K. Thomas, "Medicare Star Ratings Allow Nursing Homes to Game the System," *New York Times*, August 24, 2014, (hereafter cited as "Medicare Star Ratings Allow Nursing Homes to Game the System").

50. Thomas, "Medicare Star Ratings Allow Nursing Homes to Game the System."

51. Thomas, "Medicare Star Ratings Allow Nursing Homes to Game the System."

52. CMS Releases State Operating Manual (Appendix PP); https://www.cbdmonline.org/about-cbdm/cbdm-news/2017/07/05/cms-releases-state-operating-manual-(appendix-pp).

53. Runkle, P.V., Patient-Driven Payment Model, June 29, 2018 OHCA.

54. "Joe Biden Speaks With Meghan McCain About His Late Son Beau's Battle With Cancer"; December 13, 2017 https://www.youtube.com/watch?v=3Sa8G-VR13Q.

55. Rappleye, E. "4 Benefits of Empathy Training for Physicians" March 10, 2015, *Hospital Review*, Physician & Physician, Issues; https://www.beckershospitalreview.com/

hospital-physician-relationships/4-benefits-of-empathy-training-for-physicians.html.

56. "Searching For A Cure For Japan's Loneliness Epidemic"; https://www.huffingtonpost.com/entry/japan-loneliness-aging-robots-technology_us_5b72873ae4b0530743cd04aa.

57. Searching for a Cure for Japan's Loneliness Epidemic."

58. The Strong Robot with the Gentle Touch/RIKEN News & Media. Press Release Feb. 23, 2015 http://www.riken.jp/en/pr/press/2015/20150223_2/.

59. Brody, J. E., "The Surprising Effects of Loneliness on Health," *New York Times*, Dec. 11, 2017; www.nytimes.com/2017/12/11 well/mind/how-loneliness-affects-our-health.html.

60. https://youtube.com/watch?v=Z5fjVd65F18%3Fstart%3D6%26end%3D28.

61. Samuels, A.,"Building Better Nursing Homes," April 21, 2015; https://www.theatlantic.com/business/archive/2015/04/a-better-nursing-home-exists/390936/.

62. Atul Gawande, *Being Mortal: Medicine and What Matters in the End* (New York: Henry Holt, 2014), pp. 88–89.

63. Higgins, S & Snedegar, "Inspired by her mother, WV Woman Revolutionized Long-Term Care for the Elderly WV Public Broadcasting "Telling West Virginia's Story" December 24, 2015, *Morning Edition.*

64. "Inspired by her mother, WV Woman Revolutionized Long-Term Care for the Elderly, WV Public Broadcasting, "Telling West Virginia's Story."

65. Mallers M.H., Claver M, Lares LA. "Perceived control in the lives of older adults: the influence of Langer and Rodin's work on gerontological theory, policy, and practice," *Gerontologist*, 2014 Feb;54(1):67-74. doi: 10.1093/geront/gnt051. Epub 2013 May 30. https://www.ncbi.nlm.nih.gov/pubmed/23723436.

66. The Legend of Shahbaz, adapted from *What Are Old People*

For? How Elders Will Save the World by William H. Thomas, MD. Reprinted by permission of VanderWyk & Burnham, Acton Mass. Copyright 2004 by William H. Thomas; https://www.maine.gov/dhhs/reports/ltc-services/ShahbazLegend.pdf

67. https://en.m.wikipedia.org/wiki/GreenHouse_Project.

68. "The Green House Model: Pinnacle for Culture Change Movement." Robert Wood Johnson Foundation. http://rwjf.org/vulnerable populations/product.jsp?id=63828.

69. "Green House Project gets center stage in Capitol Hill briefings"; McKnight's. http://mcknights.com/green-house-project-gets-center-stage-in-capitol-hill-briefings/article/101278/.

70. "Call to Action: Health Reform 2009" (PDF); U.S. Senator Max Baucus (D-MT) Chairman, Senate Finance Committee; http://www.ncbcapitalimpact.org/uploadedDiles/downloads/BaucusHealthReformWhitePaper11-13-08.pdf.

71. Samuels, A. "Building Better Nursing Homes," *The Atlantic*, April 21, 2015; https://www.theatlantic.com/business/archive/2015/04/a-better-nursing-home-exists/390936/.

72. Calkins, M.P., "Powell Lawton's Contributions to Long-Term Care Settings," *Journal of Housing for the Elderly,* 17 (2008) 1-2, 67-84.

73. *Being Mortal*, p. 131

74. Louise Hay, *101 Power Thoughts* (CD).

75. Jennifer A. Brush and Rev. Katie Norris, *Getting Started with Montessori, Volume 1: Practical Life Activities for Older Adults* (Chardon, Ohio: Brush Development; 2017).

76. Roberts G, Morley C, Walters W, Malta S, Doyle C. Caring for people with dementia in residential aged care: successes with a composite model featuring Montessori-based activities. *Geriatr Nurs* 2015; 36: 106-110.

77. Sheppard CL, McArthur C, Hitzig S. A systematic review of Montessori-based activities for persons with dementia. J Am Med Dir Assoc 2016; 17:117-122.

78. Kane R.A., Caplan A.L., Urv-Wong E.K., Freeman I.C., Aroskar M.A., Finch M., *Journal of American Geriatrics Society,* 1997 Sep; 45(9):1086-93. [PubMed] [Ref list]

79. New Study Supports Chicken Soup As A Cold Remedy American College Of Chest Physicians Oct 19, 2000 *Science News* https://www.sciencedaily.com/releases/2000/10/001018075252.html.

80. Herman, C. "For Chronic Pain, A Change In Habits Can Beat Opioids For Relief April 6, 2018 Health Shots: News from NPR https://www.npr.org/.../for-chronic-pain-a-change-in-habits-can-beat-opioids-for-relief.

81. "Antipsychotic Use in Part D Enrollees with Dementia" Government Accountability Office Report, https://www.cms.gov/Medicare/Prescription-Drug-Coverage/PrescriptionDrugCovGenIn/Downloads/Antipsychotic-Use-in-Part-D-Enrollees-with-Dementia-v12092015.pdf Nov 16, 2015.

82. Jaffe, I. "GAO Report Urges Fewer Antipsychotic Drugs for Dementia Patients" Mar 2, 2015.

83. www.npr.org.

84. Jaffe, I. "Some Dementia Patients increasingly given Antipsychotics" www.npr.org/.../some-dementia-patients-increasingly-given-antipsychotics-study…May 7, 2018.

85. "'They Want Docile': How Nursing Homes in the United States Overmedicate Patients with Dementia," Human Rights Watch; https://www.hrw.org/report/2018/02/05/they-want-docile/how-nursing-homes-united-states-overmedicate-people-dementia; Feb 2015.

86. "'They Want Docile': How Nursing Homes in the United States Overmedicate Patients with Dementia."

87. Hall, A., "'I screamed, but there was nothing to hear': Man trapped in 23-year 'coma' reveals horror of being unable to tell doctors he was conscious"; Daily Mail. com, Nov. 23, 2009; https://www.dailymail.co.uk/.../

Rom-Houben-Patient-trapped-23-year-coma-conscious-a...23; Nov. 2009.

88. Serotonin: Facts, uses, SSRIs, and sources, *Medical News Today*; https://www.medicalnewstoday.com/kc/serotonin-facts-232248.

89. Brody, J.E., "The Surprising Effects of Loneliness on Health," Dec. 11, 2017, *New York Times*, Personal Health; https://www.nytimes.com/2017/12/11/well/mind/how-loneliness-affects-our-health.html.

90. Reisberg, B., Ferris, S.H., de Leon, M.J., and Crook, T. The global deterioration scale for assessment of primary degenerative dementia. *American Journal of Psychiatry*, 1982, 139: 1136-1139. https://www.fhca.org/members/qi/clinadmin/global.pdf.

91. U. Cohen and G. D. Weisman, *Holding On to Home: Designing Environments for People with Dementia* (Baltimore, MD: Johns Hopkins University Press, 1991).

92. "Governor Baker Signs Law Strengthening Alzheimer's and Dementia Treatment in Massachusetts"; 8/16/2018; https://www.mass.gov/news/governor-baker-signs-law-strengthening-alzheimers-and-dementia-treatment-in-massachusetts?_ga=2.162114814.312901268.1537123864-845005433.1537123864.

93. "Governor Baker Signs Law Strengthening Alzheimer's and Dementia Treatment in Massachusetts."

94. McAlevey, J., "The West Virginia Teachers Strike Shows That Winning Big Requires Creating a Crisis, *The Nation*, March 12, 2018; https://www.thenation.com/.../the-west-virginia-teachers-strike-shows-that-winning-big-requires-creating-a-crisis.

95. www.nursinghome411.org.

96. William H. Thomas, MD, *Life Worth Living: How Someone You Love Can Still Enjoy Life in a Nursing Home—The Eden Alternative in Action* (St. Louis: Vanderwyk & Burnham, 1996).

97. Department of Health and Human Services Centers for Medicare & Medicaid Services "Medicare and Medicaid Programs:

Regulatory Provisions to Promote Program Efficiency, Transparency, and Burden Reduction" Section 1: Proposals that Simplify and Streamline Processes paragraph p. Section 2: Proposals that Reduce and Revise Timelines, paragraphs g, h, i. Published in the Federal Register 9/20/18 CMS -3346-P the Frequency of Activities https://federalregister.gov/d/2018-19599.

98. "Medicare and Medicaid Programs; Regulatory Provisions to Promote Program Efficiency, Transparency, and Burden Reduction."

OUR LOVED ONES MATTER

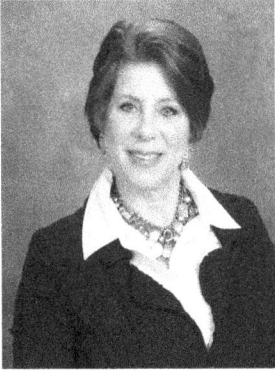

Now more than ever, you need strategies and information when considering short-term rehabilitation or long-term care needs for yourself or your loved ones.

Information is the point of power and leads you to become a more effective advocate for your loved one.

Too many times, we entrust our loved ones to a system that does not adequately or effectively care for their needs.

Phyllis Ayman has an insider's point of view, having worked in over forty skilled nursing facilities for over twenty-five years. She is also a veteran speech/language pathologist with expertise in many of the difficulties faced by older adults.

If you'd like feedback on something in particular, you can email Phyllis at: Phyllis@voiceforeldercare.com. Here you can share any experience, positive or negative, that you or a loved one is having, or has had, In the nursing home environment. Please do not include patients/ resident names or names of facilities. Feedback will be provided in forty-eight to seventy-two hours.

FREE: Download a quick 10 tip reference guide you can fill out when considering skilled nursing home placement for yourself or a loved one. Go to www.voiceforeldercare.com; you will be directed to the download page.

For more information on Phyllis Ayman's consulting services, visit
www.voiceforeldercare.com
or call 203.594.6878

www.ingramcontent.com/pod-product-compliance
Lightning Source LLC
Chambersburg PA
CBHW061024220326
41597CB00019BB/3325